"A physician is not angry at the intemperance of a mad patient, nor does he take it ill to be railed at by a man in fever. Just so should a wise man treat all mankind, as a physician does his patient, and look upon them only as sick and extravagant."

Lucius Annaeus Seneca

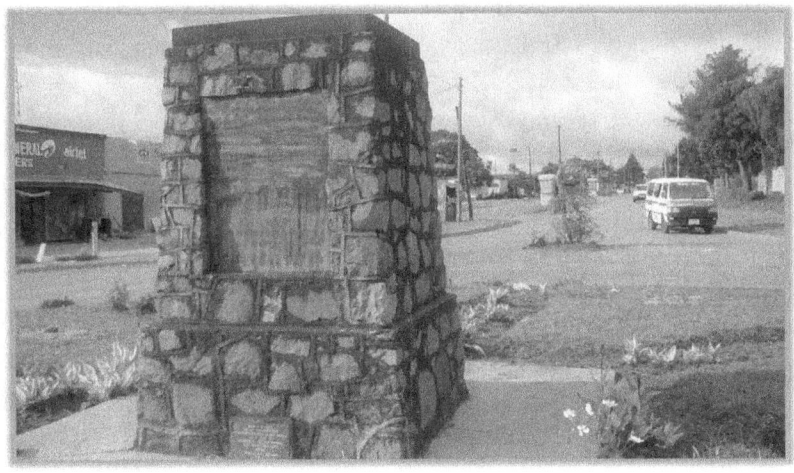

We shall defend our island, whatever the cost may be, we shall fight on the beaches, we shall fight on the landing grounds, we shall fight in the fields and in the streets, we shall fight in the hills; we shall never surrender.

Winston Churchill

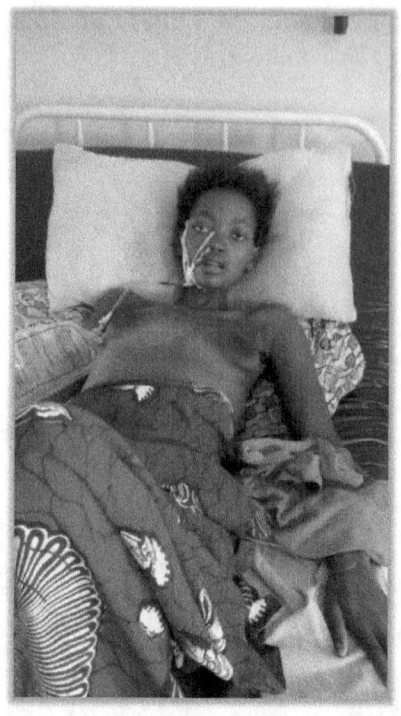

"Given one well-trained physician of the highest type he will do better work for a thousand people than ten specialists."
William J. Mayo

A Few Good Doctors

I Know What You Did in Mbala

People pay the doctor for his trouble; for his kindness they still remain in his debt.

Seneca

Inspired by a True Life Story

Dr Kelvin C Moonga

DEDICATION

This book is dedicated to my patients, past present and future.

To

Jay, John, Joshua and Matildah
whose laughter I missed dearly during the writing of this book

&

Mutinta and Victoria

My mother Pauline

For introducing me to the art of storytelling and for teaching me how to read many many years ago

My Father, J M Moonga

For his wise counsel that set me on a Career in Medicine

And

My readers for encouraging me to write this book

&

To the memory of Rhoda

INTRODUCTION

Marx is back in this epic story with fascinating drama that will leave your ribs cracked from endless laughter. While this book is a stand alone, you may be pleased to meet Marx for the first time in the book entitled, 'I know what you did in China.'

In A Few Good Doctors, Marx is trotting on home soil, in rural Zambia, doing what he loves best; caring for the sick. However, in this book, he finds himself in a very peculiar position. A social mayhem descends on his life and threatens his entire view of medical practice and passion of care.

The story is set in Mbala, an incredible town on the Northern tip of Zambia. Marx falls in love with the town's weather and its people. The community hospital where he is attached is the scene of the drama. Here, he is challenged to the deepest core of his humanity.

He knows he must remain calm in order to make sound Medical judgment on the best care his patients need. The challenges he faces threaten not only his career but the lives of his patients.

In a typical Marximillian style, he finds strength in laughter, new friendships and promise of love amidst the pandemonium taunting him.

This story is a road many have walked on and fell victim to the cruelty of men on the way. Will Marx survive the bruising conspiracy lurking in the shadows, blistering ideologies and the incredibly beautiful girls he meets?

Table of Contents

Difficult Decisions

"Doc, my sister is very sick. We want to see you. Where can we find you?" Mr. Diesel asked with audible quiver in his voice.

"Where are you?" Linda asked.

"We are on our way to the hospital," he replied.

"Take her to Fast track. You will find Dr Muhammad there. I am away from the hospital at the moment, on local leave," she replied.

Linda lay in her bed wondering what could be bothering the patient. Mr. Diesel had sounded anxious over the phone. He was a good young fellow. He was the transport officer at a local car hire and tour company, not far from Linda's Hospital, the Livingstone Royal Infirmary.

Linda had planned to spend that Saturday morning resting in bed, however she knew that call had all the tell-tale signs of calls that could ruin her off duty engagements.

It came as no surprise when Diesel called three hours later. This time he sounded extremely apprehensive in his voice.

"Doc, please allow me to come and pick you. My sister is in pain and everyone seems to be taking matters casually here. We have been sent to casualty and no one is explaining what is going on. The doctor has said my sister has a gynecological problem and we have been sent to the Radiology department. Please help me. This is my only sister," he spoke with perceptible shudder in his voice.

"Come and pick me from home," she answered reluctantly.

Diesel arrived shortly in a Metallic blue Ford Ranger. He steered the big car through Linda's small gate and brought the Ranger to a stop at Linda's front door. He killed the engine and called Linda on his Samsung galaxy cell phone. His left hand continuously tapped on the steering wheel. He held the phone in his right hand with the elbow resting on the ranger's window. The phone rang a few seconds before Linda answered.

"I am outside," he said.

"Give me a moment," she replied.

Linda emerged shortly looking gorgeous. She climbed into the ranger and immediately let her mind run through the patient's recent and past history. Mr. Diesel steered the ranger out of the gate into the main road and raced for the hospital.

"How long has she been ill?" she asked.

"I was with her yesterday till midnight. She didn't complain of anything that I know of. She was just fine. Then today, I was called at 5am that she had been taken terribly ill. She was vomiting and crying of severe abdominal pain. Then she fainted and remained powerless," Mr. Diesel explained.

They arrived at the hospital after a short drive from airport road. Linda immediately rushed to casualty to check on the patient. She found the beautiful young nurses busy with an endless flow of patients. After a brief chat, they told her the patient was sent to the Gynecology ward as the Ultra Sound Scan had reported an ovarian cyst.

Linda hurried to the gynecology ward. She got to the third floor and found several people with anxious faces lining the long Gynecology corridor. She figured these were the patient's relatives. She got to the nurses' duty room and asked for the patient's file.

"The file is still in Fast Track with Dr Mailman. I hear they are planning an evacuation to South Africa or India," the nurse on duty explained.

"I see. Where is the patient herself?" Linda asked

The nurse led Linda into the ward. They passed anxious relatives in the corridor leading to the Gyn ward. Once inside, she found the Gyn Doctors about to perform a speculum examination. The patient lay on the hospital bed disproportionately in distress. She cried where ever she was touched making physical examination misleading. Linda stood by the bed side and took a long look at the patient, observing for signs of illness that could not be exaggerated. Soon she noted the patient's abdomen was not moving in synchrony with her breathing. It appeared immobilized and rigid. She then asked the Gyn doctor, who was fighting to insert a speculum into the patient, if she could examine the patient's abdomen.

"There is nothing you find there Doc. I tried it myself. The patient is not cooperating. I am getting frustrated by her behavior. I don't like this sort of patients," Dr Inyama explained stepping aside for Linda to take over.

"Mom, my name is Linda. I would like to take a look at your abdomen," Linda asked.

"I am tired of being examined. Many doctors have examined me already and all I have received is pain. I don't want you to cause me further pain. I am tired now. Just leave me alone," the patient protested.

"Doc, just leave her, she doesn't want to be helped," the nurse retorted with exasperation visible on her face.

Linda thought for a while. She knew she had no business intruding on a Gyn case. She thought about the comfy of her bed. She could hear it beckoning her to return to it quickly. The ultra sound scan had reported that Shanelle had giant fibroids and a large cyst. Linda certainly had no business meddling with fibroids and ovarian cysts. The patient was safe in the hands of the Gynecologists. Had it not been for her unusual encounter with Little Linda at Mpelembe secondary school, an encounter that set her on a paradoxical paradigm, she would have left the ward at that very moment. She thought how worried Shanelle's brother had sounded over the phone. From her past experience caring for patients like this, she knew something was amiss. The Angel of Death could be closing in on Shanelle right under the doctors' noses. She thought against the crazy temptation brawling inside her mind to walk away from this patient. She stopped in the corridor and thought, "Why should I worry about her when they are evacuating her to India?"

"The Local air ambulance representative is here. They want to talk to Dr Mailman. May be you could talk to them," the nurse called after Linda.

"The air Ambulance crew has left South Africa; they should be landing at Livingstone international airport in 45min. The team would like to talk to a Doctor about the patient," the representative got straight to business.

"Give me a moment," she answered.

Linda walked back to the ward where Shanelle was admitted. She explained to her why she had gone there to see her. She told her how her brother had sounded worried over the phone.

"Shanelle, your brother picked me from my home to come and see you. I wouldn't be here were it not for your brother. He is worried about what could be wrong with you. I am going to examine you and inform him what I think is happening to you," Linda spoke firmly this time.

Shanelle was in her early thirties but was behaving like a teen. She turned in bed with a frown on her face and let Linda examine her. Before examining her, Linda asked which part of her abdomen was hurting the most. Shanelle pointed to the lower part on the right. And told Linda, pain had started around the umbilicus just after 4am. This information suggested Shanelle could be having appendicitis. She then turned her attention to examine Shanelle's Abdomen. She found the muscles of the abdomen rigid and a point of maximal tenderness just below the breast bone. The area over the appendix, a point known as Mc Burney's point, had increased tenderness. Linda was worried this could be due to a perforated peptic ulcer or a ruptured appendix. These diagnoses required immediate surgical intervention or the patient could rapidly change condition and die. She turned to the attending Gyn and explained.

"Doc, this is our abdomen," she said.

"What?" he asked perplexed.

"It is a surgical abdomen. Your patient has Peritonitis. She could have a ruptured Appendix or even a perforated peptic ulcer," she explained.

With these diagnoses echoing deep in her mind, she asked to talk to the Family and Mr. Diesel. The nurse quickly gathered them and led them to the nurse's station. The Air Ambulance official tagged along. Linda walked to the nurses' station wondering who this incredible patient was that had summoned an Air Ambulance to evacuate her to India. Several other doctors had gathered too, including Dr Mailman.

"Your daughter has infection in the abdomen. She has a condition known as peritonitis. She will need an operation immediately. I think this could be a complication of a perforated peptic ulcer or a ruptured appendix. I have looked at the x-rays done earlier; unfortunately they were taken with the patient supine. They have not shown us the classical picture of air under the diaphragm. We intend to re do the x-rays so that we could be certain what we are dealing with. However, that would be wasting too much time. A lot of time has been lost already. Your daughter needs immediate surgery and not further delays," she explained.

"What? An operation! That sounds too serious, doesn't it? But she was fine all day yesterday. Wouldn't giving Shanelle Injections, with strong medicines, be better than an operation?" one of the relatives remarked.

"Can that operation be done here in Zambia?" Shanelle's dad asked.

"Yes sir. Linda and her team perform this sort of operation at this hospital daily," Dr Mailman answered.

"Would you advise evacuation given what you have told the family? I have just confirmed the Ambulance is about to take off from Johannesburg," the ambulance representative asked.

"Let me put it this way; perforations of peptic ulcers carry 30% mortality rate when surgery is delayed more than seventy two hours. Like I said, our diagnosis is based purely on our clinical examination. We do not have elaborate and sophisticated testing equipment in this hospital. We use our ears, eyes and hands. I am certain this disease Shanelle has will definitely require surgery here or in India. If the surgery were to be done here, it gives her a better chance to survive because she is still stable. We do not know how much longer she has before she starts to deteriorate. I would be happy to have the surgery done right now," Linda explained.

"Papa, you have heard what the doctor is saying. The Journey to India is very long. Shanelle may not tolerate this long Journey. What do you say?" the Air Ambulance representative remarked.

"Thank you for talking to us like this. I truly appreciate what you have done. I didn't know our hospitals had doctors like you. I am deeply touched with your concerns. How long does this operation take?" Shanelle's Dad asked.

"It takes about an hour to an hour and half," Dr Ondi answered. He had been quiet, listening and evaluating the decision facing them.

"Please doctor, help our daughter. Do what you have to do," Shanelle's mom pleaded with Linda.

"Well, I guess I have to tell the ambulance crew to turn back," said the representative rising from his chair.

Linda left the room doubting her own diagnosis. The responsibilities resting on her shoulders were colossal. She was now not sure if she had made the right decision. "What if I am wrong?" she asked herself.

"Doc, do you know this family? They own that Hi Tech, multi storey shopping complex near one stop centre in down town. The elder sister is a minister at sate house. She has a brother who is a lawyer. I think he is a Judge now. They also have a brother in a senior position at Barclays Bank Plc," a short chubby lady in a black dress ran the family profile at Linda with a sardonic grin on her face.

"They are very humble people. I like them. Why are you telling me this?" she asked the sardonic lady. Linda later found out this lady was not even a family member. She was just a tag along, pretending to be friends with the family and riding on the name of this successful family.

***

Shanelle was brought into theatre shortly after the family convention. She was in obvious distress. Unfortunately, theatre had three caesarean sections from maternity and one anesthetist. They could only operate on one patient at a time. Linda's patient had to wait. However Linda was not prepared to waste another minute, her patient needed urgent surgery. She called her friend, an anesthetist scheduled to work night shift.

"Mr. Kalus, I need your help. I have a patient who needs urgent surgery. The anesthetist on duty, Mr. Kazh is overwhelmed by three Caesarean sections," she explained on phone.

"Ok I am on my way, let them take the patient inside the operating theatre," he answered without asking details about the patient's illness.

Kalus and Linda had performed countless amazing surgeries at short notice even when he wasn't on duty. Mr. Kalus was a highly competent and reliable anesthetist. He was always available at short notice. He never complained.

***

Shanelle was laid on the operating table and Mr. Kalus proceeded to put her to sleep. He intubated her and connected her to a vent.

Linda scrubbed with her assistant Dr Ondi. They draped their patient in a sterile manner using a long green theatre drape with a wide window. They dropped the head end, covering Mr. Kalus anesthetic ventilation tubing. They approached the operating table debating on which incision would be suitable to use. They settled for a midline incision.

No sooner did they enter the abdomen than they were greeted by a thick molten porridge of pus.

"Good lord, this woman is ill," Ligata the porter remarked

"And they said she only fell ill in the last six hours," Dr Ondi added.

"Is it possible for pus to form in just six hours?" Mr. Kalus asked.

"Where would one litre of pus come from in six hours? Even if it were twenty four hours, that wouldn't happen," Nurse Kapalu asked.

"Linda, did you look at her blood count results? The white cell count is very high," Tinta, a young and pretty intern doctor asked.

"I am certain she has been unwell for more than 72 hours. However, they insist she has never complained of anything in the past one month. She was at work yesterday up to midnight. If it weren't for her brother, Mr. Diesel, I wouldn't have believed the history you took," Linda explained.

Linda and Dr Ondi focused their attention to search for the source of this pus. The only sound to be heard in theatre at this point was the beeping monitors Mr. Kalus had connected to the patient and the clicking sound from the sky blue clock on the wall, two meters directly opposite where Linda stood on the operating table. A suction machine was busy sucking out the pus, ravenously, via a long straw like yellow tubing the size of a man's thumb connected to the operating table.

They found the Appendix, it looked inflamed. However it was not ruptured. It could not be the source of the pus. Next they searched the pelvic organs. They found the uterus greatly enlarged and next to it, a large corpus Luteal cyst. The Fallopian tubes, however, looked normal. They checked the entire length of small bowel starting at the ligament of Treitz. However, here too, they draw blanks.

"The uterus is very big. This is approximately 18 weeks size," Dr Ondi observed.

"If it were not for the scan Tinta requested for, I would have said she was pregnant. However the uterus is empty," said Linda.

"Shouldn't the corpus luteum grow to this size together with the uterus, in pregnancy? Do you think she could have been pregnant? I think she terminated a pregnancy and is the reason she presented late to hospital. She thought the pain had been due to an abortion even when something different had emerged. Poor girl, she would have died," Tinta postulated.

"Did you get that in your history and examination?" Dr Ondi asked.

"No I didn't. She lied about her history," Tinta defended her theory.

By now, Linda and Dr Ondi had shifted their attention to explore the stomach. Their Meticulous search was soon rewarded. They found the notorious ulcer that had perforated as Linda had suspected, hiding deep below the liver. They were certain Shanelle's killer ulcer had been perforated for more than five days. They couldn't explain why she had not complained of any pain when this happened. Perforation of peptic ulcers is a surgical emergency. Usually the patient's condition deteriorates rapidly and dies when surgery is delayed.

The next day, Linda went to the side ward in department of surgery to check on Shanelle. She found her fully alert and chatting. She was surrounded by a large circle of family members. Her brother Joe, the Attorney was there too. He had travelled over one thousand kilometers from Kitwe, to be with his beloved sister when news of her illness reached him. He wanted to know what Linda and her team found on the operation table.

"Doc, when we heard our sister had fallen ill, the whole family took to prayer. We fasted and prayed over her. I felt in my spirit, this could be an attack," He explained when they were seated in the side ward.

"We found strange things in your sister's abdomen. It can only be explained by what you are explaining to me right now. Medically it doesn't make sense, unless of course your sister lied to us. First, tell me about yourself, I am intrigued by your story," Linda started to explain.

"First, I would like to thank you for operating on my sister. I understand it wasn't easy arriving at this decision," Joe explained.

"We are grateful to the family for allowing us to operate. They placed her life in our hands and trusted our findings even when we were total strangers. We wouldn't have done anything had it not been for their permission. I found your parents extremely humble. Many families would have opted to be flown abroad for treatment. I am still surprised by the trust shown to our team by your family. Doctors can never deliver effective treatment when they leave out the family. Personally, I believe the family plays a fundamental role in patient care. I believe they form an integral unit of the care team. They are the ones that bear the hardest decision to be made. Largely because, they are asked to consent to treatment plans they may have no knowledge about. The information they are given to digest in a tense environment, took doctors more than seven years to understand. Yet families are expected to assimilate this knowledge in just a short while and consent to suggested treatments in just a few minutes. Sometimes, this is done amidst impatient health care providers. I thank your family for the difficulty decision they took yesterday. Now you can tell me about yourself," Linda explained.

"My name is Joe. I am a Pastor. I am also an Attorney. I am employed by the Judiciary in Kitwe," He explained.

"I have never met a person with such work combination. A Pastor and a Lawyer, that's an amazing calling, you carry on your shoulders. God bless you," Linda answered with deep admiration of Joe's calling.

"Thank you. My sister had a spirit that wanted to take her life. When I came into the ward this morning, I sensed it and I immediately entered into prayer and casted this evil spirit. When the evil spirit left my sister, she rose from her bed confused. She started asking where she was and what she was doing here. She was unaware she had fallen ill. Your findings in her abdomen bear testimony to this. This evil spirit would have killed my sister. God worked through you doc to make this decision to operate here. The Favour of God is upon you Dr Linda. God will make you great and lead you to higher places," He explained

"Amen," Linda answered.

This was an Amazing encounter, Doctor and Lawyer; believers in Jesus Christ. This encounter changed Linda's view about lawyers for ever. As a result of this encounter with Joe, Linda was inspired to enroll and study Law.

***

Shanelle made incredible recovery over the next few days. Five days after this incredible operation, Linda travelled to Lusaka for briefing on a trip to the Northern Province. She was very reluctant to make this trip up north.

***

When Shanelle's elder sister heard Linda was in town, she insisted they should meet. She asked Linda to spend a night at her home. She forbade her to go to a Lodge. Mr. Diesel let Linda get a vehicle of her choice from the garage where he worked. She chose the Ranger and drove thinking about Joe the Attorney and his deep love for God. She thought about God's Favour he had prophesized on her life. She left Livingstone in the early hours on Friday morning and was in Lusaka by 9am. She drove into Cairo road and found a parking space on the southern end, not far from Findeco house. There were several street boys along this once upon a time flamboyant street of Lusaka. Now, it looked dirty. The control of traffic and parking slots was left to groups of self appointed parking space vigilantes. These were often disheveled fellows, the infamous call boys of Lusaka city.

Linda got off her ranger and strode along the busy corridors of Cairo road in Lusaka. She soon disappeared into the large crowds rushing in either direction. She walked leisurely towards the northern end of Cairo road reminiscing her days as a student at great east road campus and later school of Medicine of the prestigious University of Zambia. She used to visit this street to clear her mind after weeks of none stop lectures and examinations.

At the first street turn on her left, a road leading to Kulima Tower, she ran into a doctor she had met during her last trip to China.

"Dr Maximilian, long time. How have you been?" she greeted him.

"Never been better," he answered without looking at the person greeting him. Then he looked up to see who it was greeting him. "Linda, what a pleasant surprise, what are you doing in Cairo road? Girls like you no longer come here."

"Where are they found?" Linda asked playing to be naïve.

"They are found at Levy Park, East Park, Makeni Mall, Manda hill, Arcades and Cosmopolitan or at the Emmasdale Cathedral of Blessings," he answered laughing.

"What are you doing here yourself?" Linda asked.

"I have a court case scheduled for 2pm. I am passing time talking to vendors on the streets. You will be amazed how much wisdom you can collect on street corners," he answered.

"What is the case about?" Linda probed further. She noticed Marx didn't look very happy.

"Lately, my life has generated sufficient conflict to support a million crooked lawyers," said Marx with a grin on his face. "Did I ever tell you that I was once married to a beautiful girl? This was seven years ago."

"No, you didn't," she answered curiously.

"We met at Chez Ntemba, an international night club in Cape Town. We had two wonderful children. Then she relapsed into her old ways and ran off with a stallion. This old bull could not compete with a majestic white stallion. However, hardly a year, she broke up with her deceitful Stallion. Over the last seven years she has tried to invent numerous evil schemes to hurt me. The latest was to convince the courts to take away my property. *The System* has since blocked my pay and chose to pay her instead to settle an old debt known only by her. I vowed never to engage in a legal battle with her because I knew, the law, on matters such as these, it rules in favour of women. I instead presented my case before the judge in heaven. One day the truth will be known and he will rule in my favor. I don't know what she wants this time. I will find out this afternoon," he smiled. "I think she owes a private school in tuition fees for the boys and rent. She hires many private teachers and when she can't pay, she turns to court."

"But that can't be right. Didn't she leave you on her own? Who divorced the other? By leaving on her own accord, meant she could look after herself and the kids, right. Was the court in order to give this lady your children?" she asked.

"She is so cunning that all inept legal minds easily believed her claims. I think it is her seductive sensual appeal they fall for. When you meet her for the first time, you would be certain, I was the villain. Once I was called a criminal by a dim witted divorce lawyer in a parked court room. I was so angry that I vowed to place a colostomy at the back of his neck if I ever saw that pimp in my operating theatre," Dr Marximillian explained. "She fornicates with many of these private tutors and when she is caught by their wives, she turns to me to pay for her accrued adulterous tuition fees."

"Poor woman; you are a good man. I think your war is not against flesh and blood, but principalities, authorities, demons, rulers and kings in the heavenly realms," she counseled him.

"The courts don't think so. She has been sleeping with court clerks and anything on two legs. She picks small boys to fornicate with, in the house I built for my kids. She has committed adultery with everyone previously known to me, many of whom were my close friends and then she invents ways to ensure this diabolic news of her wickedness reaches my ears. She does this in the hope that it would hurt me," Marx explained.

"Poor woman, she is only hurting herself. I think she is possessed by Satan, she needs deliverance. What went wrong with you? What were you doing picking a whore for a wife? I met a Lawyer who has inspired me into studying Law. We need this legal knowledge doc," Linda spoke with empathy in her voice. "When I graduate, hire me to be your lawyer. I will meticulously review your case and throw everyone in jail that erred in law regarding your issue. As for your ex, I'll hand her over to God's judgment. I feel sorry for her. Her end might not be pleasant, if she does not repent of her wickedness."

"It is a long sad story doc; one I would never wish for anyone. I believe children are a gift from God whether born in adultery or in a Laboratory test tube. Fortunately, they never remain children for forever. Our responsibility to them is to help them grow up and some day to become responsible independent adults. It does not matter whether they are our biological children or not; every child under the care of an adult should be treated equally; and that means, given an opportunity to grow up and acquire skills and an education necessary for survival in this sophisticated modern world. I love my children deeply. However this pretty woman, my ex, has made everyone think to the contrary. I have been to court hundred times on matters that should never come before the court," he explained with a tear in his left eye. "I pray for her deliverance daily and protection of my children. I wouldn't want the evil spirits that possess her to enter my children."

"Only love can hate and hurt like this. I feel for you doc, this must be very hard on you," she said putting her hand on his right shoulder.

"Five years before she divorced me, I watched her chase her own biological father from our house like a dog. The old fellow had come to fetch his wife that had exiled herself from her matrimonial home to our house and was now living with us. When mother and daughter saw the old folk enter our yard, they descended on him like vicious cats warding off an intruder to their den. They forbade him to enter and shut the gate to his face. I went down to check what was happening and was totally horrified to find that she was hounding her own father. When I tried to intervene, mother and daughter threatened to go and strip naked on the street if I allowed him in," Marx narrated an eerie tale.

"Abomination; you are kidding," said Linda in disbelief. "I would never disown my father in this life or the next whatever the circumstance. Isn't it written? Honor your father and mother that it may go well with you in the land. What did you do?"

"I left the angry cats and drove off with the old man. I found the words he told me on the way deeply troubling and wise. He told me a dead dog was worth more than a man without money. He was retired and penniless.

He warned me I would suffer the same fate as he at the hands of these evil women if I were not careful. He expressed deep doubt, whether my ex was his daughter at all. 'Be careful with that woman you call your wife my son,' he said. 'If she were truly my daughter, she wouldn't have chased me like a dog from your house.'" Marx recounted his eerie tale.

"Yet this is the kind of person the court gave your children to," Linda expressed profound surprise.

"When I heard these words from my in-law, I knew I could not go on living with my adorable Angelic wife. She was incapable to hold emotions of love. She was a cold blooded killer. The divorce was a welcome escape for me," said Marx smiling. "I probably might have ended up like my poor inlaw in my old age; homeless, with no one to take him to the hospital when he fell ill and only to be discovered lying on a cold murky floor dead; in a dilapidated dark room, he once called his cozy bedroom; dead like a homeless dog."

"That was the saddest and cruelest way to die for a man with grown children and a wife," she remarked on the verge of tearing. "Never marry a pretty woman. Did you know a man married to a beautiful woman has the same troubles as a man who plants his vine yard by the road side?"

"But you are a pretty woman. You are the most beautiful doctor I ever met," Marx remarked looking at Linda. "However, as I found out, beauty is a trait that is more beneficial for the women than men."

"All that glitters is not gold...," she said. "On a different note doc, I am supposed to travel to Northern Province for surgery tomorrow. Can I propose your name to the sponsors of the trip so that you travel instead?"

"I would be most delighted. I could use a break from this noise," he replied

This said, Linda bade Marx farewell and wished him God's favor and deliverance from his troubles.

***

Marx remained in Cairo road and continued talking to Vendors on the streets. Soon he ran into an interesting young man he would never forget his entire life. He sold books along the corridors. Marx got to his stand pretending to be interested in the books he sold. He then engaged the vendor into a story. His story turned out incredibly intriguing for Marx.

"Can I help you sir? Are you looking for a specific book?" the young book seller asked.

"No, thank you, I am just admiring what you do and the different books you sale," Marx answered.

"Sir, I stopped school in grade six in the village in Mapatizya, however, I can read. I have discovered that when you read a book, any book. You never remain the same. The book changes you," he explained.

"That's interesting. When you read a book, you become a different person. The book changes you. You are not the same person you where in chapter one. For how long have you been selling books," Marx asked.

"To be honest with you sir, today marks one year since I started. I started beside that tree over there," he pointed at a large Jacaranda tree in the pedestrian walk way in Cairo road. I am not a street vendor by nature. I discovered that there was a lot of money out here for any keen observer willing to learn. I started to sell on the street to learn something from the people found on these streets. Many of them are very good sales people. However many of them lack basic manners and self respect. I have tried to respect my customers all the time. I want to be different from these bozos on the street," he explained.

"How did you end up on this street from Mapatizya? What tribe are you? You speak Bemba very well," Marx asked.

"It is a long story. You must learn this; there is no tribe on the street. However, the street has one language called Money," he explained. "When you are out here, we all speak money nothing else."

"That's interesting to hear," Marx remarked.

"I learnt what I do by observing everything around me. My break came one afternoon. I was seated by that old Jacaranda tree when suddenly a man walked to my stand and started pointing at books. 'Give me that, give me that, give me that and that and that,' he said. When we counted, it came to $3,500. He pulled a large wallet and paid cash. I had to knock off that same hour fearing this man would return and bring back my books.

For two weeks thereafter, I never stopped looking over my shoulders fearing this stranger would return to demand his money back," he explained.

"Did he return?" Marx asked laughing.

"He did. Only he came for more. He got all the books I had on law. Then I asked him why he read all those law books he got. He told me knowledge of the Law was very important in the modern world. He said Law controlled all our lives. Take a doctor for instance, with all his learning; he can only work within the provision of the law. My customer worked for a Bank and wanted to protect himself by studying the law. I suggest you should study the Law too sir. If I had completed grade twelve, I would have studied Law," He explained.

Marx nearly forgot about his court case. He bought a Law book from his street friend and rushed to court.

***

Mean time that same day, Linda had visited all the places Marx had suggested to her by 5 pm. As dusk came over the city of Lusaka, she was tired and ready to visit Shanelle's elder sister. She called her host to ask whether she could have two of her best friends accompany her.

"You are most welcome my dear. It will be lovely to have company around. Your friends are most welcome too," Shanelle's sister answered in a cheerful voice on the other end of the phone.

She sounded a lovely person. She spoke as if she and Linda had met before. Linda drove to Kabwata to pick her friend Hilda and her house mate Anita. Hilda and Anita had planned to go shopping after knocking off from work. Linda had agreed to escort them to a shopping mall at Manda hill along great east road. She had not told them about Shanelle's sister. She planned to take them out on a surprised visit. The girls were delighted to see Linda after such a long while.

"Wow, you have a beautiful ride, it must have cost a fortune. Take us for a ride. We can go shopping later," said Hilda.

"No, let's go shopping. Lusaka is not good for a ride in a big car like this," Anita protested.

"I think I will just hijack you two to my hide out," Linda spoke laughing.

She drove towards city centre from Burma Road. She decided to cross Independence Avenue at the street lights and drove down to join church road. Soon they were heading towards family 24 along Lumumba road. Traffic was heavy.

"Where are you taking us doc," Anita asked with apprehension in her voice.

"This is a kidnap," Linda replied concentrating on the road.

The ranger was soon cruising through Lusaka west and the girls looked worried.

"Where are you taking us doc?" Hilda asked with audible worry in her voice.

"You are scared; I have a surprise for you. You are safe, don't worry," Linda tried to reassure the girls.

Anita stared through the window with her hands supporting her chin. She was visibly uninterested in this unplanned road trip towards a mysterious destination. After an anxious 30min drive the ranger came to a stop in front of a huge black gate. Linda pulled her cell phone and made a call. As soon as she put her phone down, the large gate opened automatically. Linda guided the ranger along a beautiful drive way towards an elegant large country house with a green tiled roof. Several beautiful cars were parked in the yard; a white Range rover sport, a BMW 5 series, a Mercedes ML 450, and some other pretty cars. The lawn looked pretty all around the house. An elegant swimming pool adorned the back of the house not far from a beautifully thatched bar.

"What is this place doc?" Hilda asked perplexed.

"Wow, it is very beautiful. People live like this in Zambia. Looks like we have travelled out of Zambia," Anita commented walking cautiously behind Hilda.

While they were absorbing the surrounding, the front door opened and a gorgeous lady in her mid thirties came out to meet them. She had a wide pleasant smile on her face. The girls immediately loved her.

"Welcome my sisters. Welcome to my humble home. Come on inside," she said.

She led them into a large and gorgeous living room. Beautiful chandelier hung from the ceiling from where the light came from. They sparkled beautifully onto a shine tiled floor. There were several elegant leather sofas facing two large flat screen television sets.

"Welcome home. Please make yourselves comfortable," their host beckoned the visitors to take seats.

"This is Hilda, she is a Pharmacist," Linda introduced her friend.

"Welcome Hilda, I am pleased to meet you. Feel at home," she answered.

"This is Anita; she is an environmental health scientist. She works for University Hospital,"

"Welcome Anita, How do you do?"

"How do you do mom?" Anita answered.

"Feel at home," she said with a warm smile.

"Finally, I am Linda, we spoke on the phone," said Linda laughing.

"Linda, I am short of words to thank you. Thank you for saving my sister."

While Linda and Shanelle's sister discussed the operation Linda had performed, Anita and Hilda asked to run around and admire the house. They had never been inside a house as elegant as this one.

They entered the kitchen and where completely won over by it. A large intelligent fridge welcomed them into the kitchen. A hefty stove with a mysterious over head canopy beckoned them to cook dinner on it. It had a transparent upper surface and numerous strange buttons on its glassy awning. The girls had never seen anything like it before. Anita and Hilda stared at this incredible kitchen in attar amusement. Next to the sink, an enchanting gas stove too, beckoned the girls to light it and fix dinner on it. On their right, a large walk in pantry, the size of a master bedroom blew their minds off. A large window opened to a beautiful car park where elegant cars rested their sporty wheels. The girls lost all sense of time as they explored this magnificent restaurant. Linda followed to fetch them seeing they had been gone for a long while.

"Are you ok in here?" she asked when she got into the kitchen.

"Linda, would you look at this marvelous kitchen? It is more expensive than my father's entire house," said Anita visibly fascinated.

"Ask your friend to allow us to cook dinner for you," said Hilda emerging from exploring the walk in storeroom.

"She has left. She has been called for an emergency meeting at state house. We are alone now. She said, it is our house and we should be free and enjoy ourselves," said Linda smiling.

"You are kidding us. This is better than being at a five star hotel," Hilda answered.

"I want to jump into the swimming pool after dinner. There are a lot of large sausages in the Fridge. I want to have sausage," said Anita.

"I have never seen sausage this big and beautiful. I could even eat it raw. I call them juicy sausages," said Hilda walking towards the colossal fridge.

"Hope you carried your swimming costume," said Linda smiling.

"You said we are alone, I want to swim naked under the moonlight. I want to make this hijack, the most memorable week end I ever had in Lusaka west," Anita answered laughing.

The girls slept late that Friday night. They could not thank Linda enough for taking them on an unexpected Lusaka weekend out. They were determined to spend their weekend at this gorgeous Palacio Hacienda and create memories that would last a life time.

The Long Way Up

Marx had a long Friday night. His court case had not gone well. He couldn't wait to take the long journey up north, far away from his troubles. While the girls where fixing themselves English breakfast at the Hacienda in Lusaka west, Dr Marximillian arrived at Lusaka intercity bus terminus. He was horrified at its appearance. The place looked deplorable and wild. In his mind, this place was supposed to be a show case of his country's beauty and hospitality. He wondered at the thoughts of foreign travelers to Zambia passing through this piece of junk. Marx was convinced the term intercity was a misdemeanor. He wished the managers of Levy Junction could take over management of this eye sore and turn it into a gem in the heart of town. Marx was convinced the appearance of a public place reflected the kind of clientele it attracted and thriftiness of its managers.

After buying his ticket, Marx decided to take a stroll to Zambia Centre for Accountancy Studies just opposite the intercity bus terminus before ending up at Levy Junction, a majestic and prosperous shopping mall. He walked along church road to central police and finally visited Evelyn Hone College. He was appalled at the paradox he uncovered. He wished he could meet the bosses of the five institution located in the same area of town yet so far apart on the development scale. Marx was convinced a century of development separated Levy Junction from intercity. This short leisurely walk had given him a sense of time travel and left him wondering what his journey up north had in store for him. He missed Guangzhou south railway station. He was convinced he would be ashamed to bring his Chinese girl friend, Liu Lu, through this station.

***

Marx chose seat number four on the Judean Luxurious coach. He sat next to a young man, a teacher in his late twenties. They exited the congested station at 2pm and drove into intercity Avenue. They passed the magnificent Zambia Centre of Accountancy studies and drove slowly towards the flamboyant Levy Junction to join church road. Traffic was heavy at the fly over bridge right up to the junction with Cairo road. Marx stared out through the window at the old post office building on his left and then looked at the magnificent Farmers' park to his right. The unsolved paradox he had grappled with earlier came to hound his brain all over again.

As Marx thought over management issues of public infrastructure and public finance, the driver steered his big golden orange scania bus into Cairo road and cruised towards Kabwe round about. They had entered T2, a transit lane referred to as the Great North Road. Marx wondered whether the proposed grade twelve certificate in the new constitution, as a minimum qualification necessary for someone to hold public office would sieve out the stubborn chuff in the public service and provide void management structures with an elite pool of skilled personnel to drive development and rival that at magnificent city stations in Europe; Civil Engineers, Architects, City planners, Public Finance managers and City Mayors at Master degree level from Top Ranked Universities in the World. Marx concluded his paradoxical enquiry and solved his polynomial by factoring out the weed and the chuff.

He leaned back in his chair and was about to doze off when the teacher seated next to him started talking to him.

"Debt is the most terrible trap a man can get caught up in," he said. Would you like to hear my story?"

"Sure, I could use a good tale. The journey ahead is long; 1000 km," he answered.

"I have been on this Great North Road numerous times. I think it is marked T2 on satellite maps. At this speed, I will arrive in Kasama tomorrow around 3am," said the teacher

"What! Tomorrow; and when do I arrive in Mbala?" Marx asked as Lusaka town faded away behind them.

"Mbala; from Mpika, you will leave Great North Road and take the M1 road. If you want to arrive early, you have to forget about arriving in the first place. These buses usually arrive in Mbala around 5am," he answered.

"That's fifteen hours of travelling. Not even a Trans Atlantic flight takes that long. A flight to Baiyun international airport in Southern China from KK takes thirteen hours. What's wrong with this country?" bemoaned Marx. He looked out of the window and admired the beautiful savannah grasslands they were driving through.

"A flight from Lusaka to Cairo in Egypt is only five to six hours. And yet we have to travel for fifteen hours from Lusaka to Mbala. Our transport system sacks. It is still very primitive," the teacher complained. The bus squeaked and roared on the narrow road ahead.

"I wonder how long it used to take before these roads where tarred. I guess people used to travel at the back of Lorries in those days. We are better off in this luxurious coach even though the journey is long," Dr Marx consoled his colleague.

They passed several truck and trailers loaded with copper destined for export in its raw form. Traffic was heavy towards Chisamba, a beautiful farming block located between Lusaka and Kabwe. The locals sold a variety of farm produce along the highway. Marx admired the succulent water melons sold at several road side markets they drove past.

"We are fortunate we got on this bus where everyone looks civilized and business executive like. There are days when you aren't so luck and have to use an old bus with an obnoxious interior. This journey can be an endless persecution on some buses," the teacher reiterated Marx worst nightmare about public transport.

"It is no wonder planes and some trains are fitted with 'first class' compartments," said Marx. "This driver shouldn't be chatting on phone like that."

Seated in his croaky chair by the window, Dr Marximillian witnessed several violations of traffic rules, both from within and without. The driver talked endlessly with his co-driver at the front and hardly kept his eyes on the road. Marx thought the driver ought to be concentrating on the road ahead. He didn't like this bus driver at all. He had just broken several traffic rules including using his cell phone and speaking endless on phone most of the way whilst driving on the busy highway. He made Marx very anxious. This highway was notorious for some of the most horrific road traffic accidents involving trucks and buses.

"This is the kind of drivers you have to put up with on this route. Some are extremely rude when you try to correct them," Daliso agreed with Marx's consternation. "You know I used to be opposed to these social partitions when I was in college. I saw them as tools to segregate the poor from the rich. These long journeys changed my mind. On one such trip north, I shared a seat with a person lacking in basic manners, my tribal cousin. She was what I would call a hag, a very unpleasant old woman. She made my journey so miserable that I had to get off the bus in Mkushi. She had carried some strange smelly food and as if that was not enough, she kept buying food at every station the bus stopped and chewed it in the most annoying demeanour I have ever seen."

The teacher narrated his ordeals on this route with earnestness on his face. They had passed the historic town of Kabwe and where now heading towards Kapiri Mposhi town. This next town was once famous and home to Zambia's glass industry. Unfortunately, like many industries in Zambia, Kapiri Glass died in its infancy. They came to a Toll gate, the first Marx had seen in his country, before driving through a weigh bridge. There were several trucks lining up, waiting their turn at the weigh bridge. Marx wondered at the basic qualification required for someone to work at the toll gate and weigh bridge. The bus was delayed by 45 minutes in Kapiri before being allowed to continue on its long journey North.

In Mkushi, everyone got off the bus to stretch their weary legs. The drivers exchanged seats. Marx and Daliso Banda the teacher got off to fetch some refreshments at a fast food take away, in front of a service station.

Marx couldn't stop thinking about the poor woman Daliso had talked about. He felt sorry for her. He thought she gorged herself in this manner due to an anxiety disorder. He thought Daliso had judged her too harshly. She was just an innocent patient who probably resorted to indiscriminate food indulgencies in order to compensate for her phobia and anxiety of long distance travel. Dr Marximillian gave her a working diagnosis of

Great North Stress and Anxiety Disorder, *GNSAD*. He was sure; he would have prescribed an anxiolytic for her had he sat next to her. He wondered how she would look like on a 600 Seater Airbus A800 or Boeing 747, Rolls-Royce Turbofan-powered wide body commercial passenger plane, cruising at top speed of *Mach 0.89*, far above the clouds on a seventeen hour Trans Atlantic Flight.

By now, it was night fall in the small town of Mkushi and the temperature plummeted. From there on, it would be a long cold ride up north. Fortunately, Daliso kept Marx busy with his tales.

"I am stuck at a rural school owing to a stupid loan I took," Daliso started talking when the bus drove off.

"Hope it wasn't a loan to buy the Ark or the Alpaya *(Alteza)*," Marx remarked.

"How did you know?" Daliso asked surprised.

"I don't know why teachers love that dangerous family bus. The Noah and its evil cousin the '*Al paya*' have annihilated lots of families you know. Friends of mine call the Alteza, *the 'WM* short for Widow Maker," Marx explained.

"I used it for business during my trips to Lusaka. The space allowed me to carry passengers on the road to meet my fuel costs. I was studying for my degree by distance Education at Rusangu University in Monze," Daliso explained.

"Cost sharing ah..," said Marx looking at the road ahead through the driver's window. Just then, a rugged looking bus named Taqua overtook them as though they were stationary.

"There goes Taqua. It runs with the wind," Daliso remarked.

"I remember seeing this bus at intercity in Lusaka. We left it at the station. What speed is it doing?" Marx remarked as the Taqua's tail lights faded and disappeared in the distance. "So what happened to your Noah?"

"I was happy the first six months. I made my journeys to school in style. My Fuel expense was met by the passengers I picked on the way. Occasionally I raced with the Taqua buses. One day I was not so lucky. I had taken a few beers to keep me awake on the road. It happened so fast. I just remember waking up in a hospital with a tube in my chest and a mangled limb," said Daliso looking at an ugly scar on his right wrist. "I was breathing through a tube in the intensive care unit. They told me I had suffered head injury even when I saw no wounds on my head."

The bus rumbled on and squeaked gracefully along the narrow patch of tarred earth stretching endlessly in the night. The bus sliced through the darkness relentless on the road ahead. There was nothing great Marx saw about this endless rugged dark void. The second driver had now taken charge of their bus and firmly kept his eyes on the road ahead. With aching Achilles tendon in his right leg, he kept his foot on the gas untiringly. His large left hand rested on the gear stick ready to change the gears whenever his twelve cylinder engine made the demand. It was as if, the road had hypnotized him. Marx did not envy his job at all; however, he respected it a great deal. He had their lives in his hands.

The two travelers chatted on. Several other passengers were engrossed in their own chitchats at various points of the bus.

"The good thing you are alive," Marx consoled Daliso.

"Unfortunately, I wasn't so smart. As soon as I was out of hospital, I went to get more loans to repair my Ark. I had a Loan from an Evil Bank and Asshole Finance. Before I knew it, I was trapped and wallowing inside a Debt prison. For the past five years, I couldn't move out of the village. I was stuck while these financial institutions merciless took my money away. I had to put my studies on hold as a result. You will be shocked at how many teachers and nurses are stuck in the villages owing to these knee jerk loans. I lived on a slave wage for the past five years," Daliso lamented.

Marx's mind slithered into deep thoughts while Daliso slipped into a snooze. He began to think of how to make this trip up north in a more civilized manner. 'One thousand kilometers on a bus is loutish to a 21st century traveler, unless that trip was a site seeing road voyage by a bunch of delusional tourists,' he murmured.

Marx was convinced a Bullet train was the perfect solution for such a long journey. He reminisced the glorious moments he had on a bullet train in china from Guangzhou in Guangdong province to Wuzhou with his Chinese girl friend, Liu Lu. Wuzhou is located in eastern Guangxi bordering Guangdong province. Marx was certain, the bullet train could reduce this horrendous 16 hours trip to just a 2 hour excursion.

He wondered what curse had befallen Africa and his country in particular as he thought about the Train a` Grande Vitesse (TGV), France's high speed rail service. Marx remembered seeing a news headline, announcing a record for the fastest wheeled train, reaching 574.8 km/h on 3rd April, 2007. In mid 2011, scheduled TGV trains operated at the highest speeds in conventional train service in the world, regularly reaching 320km/hr.

These thoughts were not a figment of Dr Marximillian bored mind on a long slow persecutory journey. Following the commercial success of the first Ligne a` Grande Vitesse (LGV), French for High Speed Line; a line centered around Paris, France's neighboring countries; Italy, Spain and German emulated this service and developed their own high speed rail services. The TGV system itself extends to France's neighboring countries and even links Britain.

While trains were going faster and faster everywhere in the world, they were getting slower and slower in his country. Recently, his country had launched a train named after the country's latest late president. Marx wondered what this train's top speed was. He was certain a Kenyan marathon splinter could out run it.

Marx wondered how a ride on the Shanghai Maglev would feel like. This is a Magnetic Levitation Train that operates in Shanghai, China. The top operational commercial speed of this train is 431 km/hr, making it the world's fastest train in regular commercial service since 2004. The Chinese Maglev has a length of 153m, a width of 3.7m, a height of 4.2m and a three class, 574 passenger configuration.

It was clear; this would be a long journey for Dr Marximillian Mukonka Chiti. His journey on the Great North road was far from being a great north ride. He wished he could build his own Great North Maglev and cruise through this remoteness in just two hours.

In Serenje, Daliso decided to get off the bus. He gave no reasons for getting off here and Marx chose not to intrude in his privacy. "A man got to go when he needs to go," he murmured to himself. He bid Marx farewell and disappeared in the cold night outside. When Marx returned to his seat, he found a pretty young lady had taken it.

"I hope I haven't taken your seat," she asked seeing he was looking at her. Marx's quick mind fumbled to find an appropriate response.

"As a matter of fact, yes but you can have it. Where is a pretty young lady heading to in the middle of the night?" he asked taking Daliso's seat.

"Thank you, I love sitting next to the window on these buses. I enjoy looking out of the window. I am going to Mpulungu to visit my sister," she answered.

"It is nearly midnight and cold outside," Marx struggled for words to keep the flame of the conversations going.

"It's the only way if I have to arrive early. This bus will be in Mpulungu at five or six. It will be perfect for me. I can finish my business and return same day with the 12 hours bus from Mpulungu. I may use this same bus," she smiled gorgeously at him.

She wore a sweet perfume that made Marx's heart race inside his chest. His general blood circulation improved to every organ in the body and all the appendages on his body. Sleep left him at once. The gods had been kind on him by sending this night angel. Although Marx was skeptical of all ladies that had no fear of the night, he was willing to make an exception on this one.

"I am Marx," he introduced himself. "This is my first trip to Mbala."

"Pleased to meet you Mr. Marx, I am Nakazwe Isaacs," she answered.

"It is Dr Marximillian but you could call me Marx," he said hoping to improve his leverage.

"So you are a Doctor," she paused thinking of her next sentence.

Marx didn't want to spoil the conversation by turning it into a medical consultation. He was afraid she might consult him on some horrendous illness she suffered from.

"I am a doctor for fish. Not humans. I work for the Fisheries department. I am on a quest to check out some unique fishes in Lake Tanganyika," he smiled. "So… Isaacs; your dad's or spouse…?"

"My dad's; he was Irish. Mom met him in Mbala. I have never met him," she answered looking down as the bus came to a stop in Mpika.

Marx didn't notice the nearly 300km distance between Serenje and Mpika. He was sure Daliso had slowed down the bus earlier. His debt was too heavy on the bus. Isaacs had changed the speed. He thought these things as he got out of the bus to look for the Men's convenience. Blood flow to his kidneys had improved and the bladder was beginning to fill rapidly. At that moment, he would have refused to trade his Stone Age bus ride for a Shangai Maglev.

He returned to the bus carrying two disposable cups of coffee. He passed one to Ms Isaacs as he sat down.

"Coffee," he said.

"Wow, thank you, I love coffee," Her eyes brightened up as she got the cup from his big hand.

In Mpika, the bus turned off the great north road they had travelled all this while on to a narrow tarred road, M1. Marx didn't like the look of this small road. Isaacs noticed the look on Marx face.

"This road goes to Mpulungu. It will now take us to Kasama. It is a three to four hour drive from here. The road we have left goes to Tanzania. It is the Great North Road," she explained sipping her coffee.

"You read my thoughts," he said.

"As a matter of fact yes," she giggled. "Sometimes I read people's minds."

"Can you read my next thoughts?" he asked.

"Mm, let's see," she turned in her chair and faced him. She looked him straight in the eye. "You are divorced and in debt. You are kind of lonely too."

Marx burst out laughing and spilled some coffee on his lap. "You are cruel. That is very true, how did you know this? I hope it is not written all over my forehead."

"You are too generous, you surrendered your seat to me a midnight stranger; you look mid thirties and are handsome. You are travelling alone in the middle of the night too," she answered with her head tilted to an angle towards her left shoulder smiling. She read him like a book.

"I think you are a Psychologist or Psychic. Where do you work?" Marx was curious.

"I help people incarcerated by the four evil sisters; Debt, Divorce, Disease and Death," she said calmly.

"Divorce, Debt, Disease and Death," Marx repeated the notorious 'D' words thoughtfully. "Is there anything one can do to save the Dead? Only the living can be helped."

"I work for the Credit Reference Bureau, CRB, in Lusaka. Our offices are near the intercity bus terminus. You should bring me some fish one day," she smiled and stared out through the window.

"CRB… what is the credit burden for Zambians now?" he asked changing the subject from psychoanalysis and the infamous evil quartet. He was sure she already knew what was on his mind.

"People are in deep trouble with debt Marx. I deal with difficulty clients; many come to shout at us in the offices for listing them down," she explained.

"That must be bad," he said.

"I remember this one file I was working on; the client's name was given to us by his bank. He had defaulted on his loan for six months. I called his cell to arrange a meeting. His nephew answered the phone and told me his uncle had a stroke and that he could not talk. When I called a month later, I was told he had died," she explained.

"What do you do in cases like those?" He asked.

"We ask the next of kin to submit hospital records, death certificates or a coronus report in cases of death outside the hospital," she explained.

"That explains a lot of things now; when I was a young medical doctor, straight from university; we used to have several people coming to our hospital asking for replacement of lost death certificates for deceased relatives. Some people would even offer money for a death certificate. Once I was offered $10,000 to write a death certificate for a living person," Marx explained recalling spurts of death certificate forgeries that had become rampant at his hospital.

"You said you are a Fish doctor, didn't you?" Isaacs asked suspiciously at Marx

"Jesus told his disciples he would make them Fishers of Men," Marx answered and smile warmly at her. They laughed candidly together. She let him hold her hand.

The bus drove into the next city majestically. Gospel music played from inconspicuous speakers on the bus. Marx had noticed this practice by most bus crews. It was hoped a serene church atmosphere could cast away evil spirits from the bus and guarantee a safe passage through some haunted spots on the road.

Road traffic accidents, involving buses, had increased in the recent months. The travelling public was gripped with fear. It was 3am in Kasama and Marx had been awake for forty two hours. He considered spending the rest of that morning with Ms Isaacs. He was worried their friendship had matured too fast. It had no real structures supporting it. It reminded him of his Chez Ntemba escort. He was still suffering the consequences of that horrible Cape Town mess.

The journey from Mpika to Kasama had only taken '3 Isaacs'. This was his new way of counting the passage of time. He was certain Kasama Mbala would take only 'a half Isaac'. He didn't have much time left. She had told him he was lonely. This Journey had quadrupled his lonesome rating. He wished he had a flower and pluck out its petals to help him arrive at a decision.

"Should I tell her? I should tell her not, Should I tell her? I should tell her not," he thought to himself plucking petals from an imaginary purple flower.

"You have gone quiet on me. I guess I talk too much or maybe you are too tired…," she teased him seeing he had slipped into deep thought.

"I enjoyed your company very much. You made this long journey appear very short," he answered. "You made it seem like I took a Bullet train to Mbala."

"I am fluttered. Most people find me boring. They say I am too proud," she said taking his hand in hers.

"You are the most exciting person I have met. If I had my own way, I would never want you to leave my side. I would take you to the hospital so that a surgeon would stitch us together at the head," he said resting her hand in his.

"Really and be turned into Siamese twins," she smiled. "We have only met but I feel I have known you for years.

"We would become what are known as craniopagus twins," he smiled.

The bus entered Mbala and drove up President Avenue. It circled the war memorial monument and came to a stop at Arms Hotel, an old building with imposing British architecture. Marx had arrived at his final destination.

He sat in his chair struggling to tear himself from his craniopagus twin. Ms Isaacs' charm was too strong to resist. After a long internal battle, he decided it was for the best that he let his mysterious girl friend proceed on her way.

"Aren't you going to invite me in," she asked when the bus came to a stop.

"I snore like a million pigs. You would run away in the middle of the night," he answered smiling. "Maybe when I am in Lusaka, you could invite me."

"You should come and see me in Lusaka," she said with disappointment in her voice. "Enjoy Fishing in Mbala."

He was aware, evil lurked at every corner looking for someone stupid to devour.

"In the weird world today, demons too could take the bus," he murmured as he stepped out of the bus.

Hit the Ground Running

Marx awoke at 1pm at Triple Palm Lodge. He was hungry and anxious to tour his new home. He took a quick shower and emerged from his room feeling rejuvenated. It was raining outside. April looked so beautiful out here. He could sense the month in the air. He stood at the front of his little Lodge and took a long deep breath. He filled his lungs with fresh air around him. He immediately fell in Love with Mbala town and its wonderful people. He was certain he would enjoy his stay and use the time to reflect.

Everywhere he looked, the vegetation was green. The trees looked beautiful. Triple Palm Lodge was built overlooking a small river famous for its palm trees that grew in it. Marx gazed upon in awe. The enchanting large palm trees stretched in the distance as far as the eye could see. They run with the river its entire course. The impression it gave Marx was as if he were viewing a biblical city.

While he gazed on the river, a waiter came to tell him his Lunch was ready in the restaurant. After a scrumptious Lunch of Nshima with Fish, Marx was taken for a tour of Abercorn Community Hospital. A doctor came to pick him in his private car.

***

"Welcome to Mbala Dr Marximillian. I hope you had a wonderful trip," said Dr Kalunda reaching out to greet Marx.

"I enjoyed my Journey very much. I can't wait to see your hospital," Marx answered.

"You are sure you are not tired," Dr Kalunda asked when they were seated in the car.

"I am as fit as a fiddle," he replied.

"Very well then, let's go to the hospital. Actually, I have a patient we kept for you. We wanted to refer her to Kasama. When I heard you were coming, I kept her for you to see." Kalunda explained.

They drove for the hospital on a bumpy gravel road. Marx noted the soils to be red all around. The houses and buildings he saw were stained with red mud on their walls. Red dirty could be seen trapped on many windows and roofs he saw. This gave him a glimpse into the blistering winds that pounded the town in the dry months of the year. He would not experience these winds as this was the rainy season in Mbala.

The weather was cool, a kind of weather Marx loved. A drizzle persisted since morning and made the gravel road slippery even for off road vehicles. The hospital road presented a treacherous bumpy ride.

"Your roads are very bad," said Marx when their car came to a notoriously bumpy stretch.

"These roads have been neglected for a long time. Fortunately they will be worked on starting next month. The contractor is already on site. A Chinese company was awarded a contract to do the roads," Dr Kalunda explained as they drove into the hospital grounds.

Abercorn Community Hospital was built on elevated ground. To a casual observer, the hospital looked as though it had been built on a hill side. The civil engineers and landscapers had created an illusion of a hospital built on a hill side. It was a beautiful little health facility. Its Façade was adorned by numerous indigenous trees as well as exotic ones. Their ever green canopies towered high above the cars in the parking lot.

Dr Marximillian recognized Acacia Albina, Vitex Doniana, Umufungo and several exotic Pine trees. This beautiful tree garden reminded him of his freshman year and of his professor of plant biology in the school of Natural Sciences. The lawns were well kept and incredibly green. Marx followed his host along a wide walk way that rose at a fifteen degree incline. They turned left and entered a wide corridor that stretched far in the distance. They made a right turn immediately after entering this colossal corridor.

"This is our Maternity ward doc," Dr Kalunda explained.

"You have a beautiful hospital," Marx replied admiring this little community hospital.

They passed several side wards on their right and soon entered the main ward at the far end. Rhoda, the patient kept for Marx lay on a bed at the back of the ward. She was visibly very ill. Flies of different sizes never left her bed side. An awful reek rose from the bed on which she lay. Marx's big heart immediately went out to her. He wanted to do something immediately.

"We admitted Rhoda one month ago as a referral from Mpulungu, for septic abortion. She has had two laparotomies but has not shown any improvement. She has deteriorated over the past two weeks. I kept her for you. I know you will help her," Kalunda explained.

A thought began to form inside Marx's mind. "Doc, why do you hate me so much? What have I done to you to deserve such a hopeless case like this? You should have sent her away," he thought to himself.

He turned to examine the patient. The reek coming out of her hospital beddings could kill a man. Marx found himself feeling sick. He requested for gloves and gave her a thorough examination.

They left the Gynecology ward and toured other sections of the hospital, beginning with the pediatrics department, then medicine and psychiatry. Throughout the tour, Marx could not rid his mind of Rhoda. The reek from her bed kept coming at him. He could see her frail face and faint eyes begging him to save her. He found himself regretting accepting Linda's work.

After, a long hospital tour, the host doctor decided to take his visitor for some refreshments on the shores of Lake Chila. They drove through the small town of Mbala, and crossed it in a matter of minutes. Several shops, with fancy names, where doted all along the side of the road. At the far end of President Avenue, they passed a large blue building on the left. Marx recognized the premises and was certain this was the main police station of Mbala town. While he was still admiring the building, a white motor bike with an attached passenger cabin on its left side veered in through the gate. Marx last saw these scooters in German war movies and world war documentaries. He was certain; someone had fished this one out of Lake Chila. He had read somewhere that after Germany surrendered during world war one, the German troops stationed in Mbala were ordered to throw their weapons and military hardware into lake Chila. He couldn't wait to see this infamous Lake, where fish swam with Landmines, Bombs, Sub Machine Guns and Tanks. He wondered how fish from this lake tasted. The prospects that the Lake could be mined did not please Marx. By now, dusk was hovering over the small town of Mbala and the temperature plummeted. Marx was beginning to freeze.

***

Later in the evening he returned to his lodge still thinking about Rhoda. She had had two operations already. He wasn't sure whether a third would save her life. She was severely anemic, with a Hemoglobin count of 5g/dl. He was sure; it would take a miracle to save Rhoda. While he thought these things, he decided to shift and move to a more tranquil lodge in town. He considered moving to a lodge along the shores of Lake Chila.

He checked himself at Giza Inn. The rooms looked cozy and met with his basic standards for lodging. Marx's sharp medical mind took a quick survey of room 12B. A study desk was placed next to a mahogany wardrobe, coffee making facilities sat next to a small fridge just below a wide flat TV screen mounted on the wall at the foot end of a Queen Size bed. He didn't like the bed. He was sure it harbored numerous evil secretes. He wondered how many sins had been committed on it by immoral guests before him. If sin was contagious, he was sure that night would leave him morally ill. He couldn't bring his mind to list the kind of sins people committed on beautiful beds like the one in his room. He wished he could request for a disposable bed. There was no air-conditioning unit on the wall. He wasn't sure he would need it. Giza was a small tranquil resort in mbala central business area hidden from plain view of a casual traveler. This would be Dr Marximillian home during his short stay in Mbala.

Dr Marx sat on his bed still thinking about Rhoda. By now, it was 8pm in Mbala. He decided to take a hot shower. Hardly five minutes into his cozy shower than his phone rang. It was the hospital.

"Dr Marximillian, this is the coverage nurse. I got your number from Dr Kalunda. We have just admitted a patient with suspected intestinal obstruction, a referral from Mpulungu hospital. The doctor on call is requesting for your opinion as there is no blood in the hospital," a male nurse, with a fun accent, explained.

"Send transport to pick me at Giza Inn. I am in room 12B," he answered.

Dr Marx dried himself quickly and dressed hurriedly. He had not had supper. And suddenly he was feeling hungry. He quickly made himself coffee and opened a pack of biscuits. He thought about the worst case scenario; gangrenous compound sigmoid colon volvulus was top on his list together with a gangrenous ceacal volvulus. He was sure to be gone for a very long time if he was faced by any one of these killer afflictions.

The driver arrived shortly. They drove to the hospital in a landcruiser along the bumpy road he and Dr Kalunda had used earlier that day. He bounced up and down in the passenger seat. The empty chairs at the back rattled endlessly to the hospital.

He alighted at the entrance to the administration block and speeded for the operating theatre. The Doctor on call had decided to book the patient for immediate surgery and went back to his house to continue with his sleep.

Marx was met by the coverage nurse that had made the call. He was a serious looking young fellow whom Marx liked immediately. Several nurses and students were there to watch the visiting doctor stumble with his first major case at Abercorn.

Marx emerged from the male change room and hurriedly found his way through the maze of the colossal theatre. He deeply loved this Abercorn theatre. There was enough space for a dozen to play hide and seek. He found the patient, a young man in his early twenties, had already been placed on the operating table. He was in obvious distress and deeply jaundiced. Marx proceeded to examine the patient's abdomen. What he found surprised everyone.

"This patient has peritonitis," he announced to the anxious onlookers. "I will need a minimum of twelve litres of normal saline to wash his abdomen."

"We only have two litres of Ringer's lactate in theatre," the theatre nurse announced.

"Coverage, get me ten litres of saline before I wash your patient's abdomen with tap water," he answered. "Nurse, you can start scrubbing, I will join you shortly."

"Can we move the patient to the dirty cases theatre since you are saying it is now peritonitis?" the theatre nurse asked.

The anesthetist watched quietly at the drama in theatre. He and Marx had met before. He proceeded to put the patient to sleep as soon as the team was ready. The coverage nurse emerged shortly with a pint of blood and ten litres of saline.

Dr Marx hastily approached the operating table after being gowned in a long green priestly robe. He cleaned the patient's abdomen with three different solutions the theatre nurse passed to him in a ceremonial manner. He then covered the patient, with the help of the theatre nurse head to toe. The abdomen could be seen through a window in the abdominal drape they used.

At 10pm, the operation was finally under way. Dr Marx cut through the skin from the sternum down to the pubis symphysis. Once inside the abdominal cavity, he was greeted by two litres of pus.

"You see why I wanted twelve litres of saline," he said looking at the coverage nurse who had stayed to watch the operation.

"I see doctor," he answered.

"But why so much fluid, can't you just suck out the pus using the suction machine. We have serious shortages of fluids in this hospital," the theatre nurse offered an argument.

"My dear nurse, the outcome of this disease is directly proportional to how thorough you washed the abdomen during surgery. I reviewed a patient, called Rhoda in Maternity. She has had two operations and she is going to have a third one tomorrow. Do you know why?" Marx asked looking at the theatre nurse.

"No. Maybe her immune system is weak," she answered.

"She is coming because you washed her abdominal cavity with only one litre of Ringer's Lactate. She was inadequately treated. She now has tertiary peritonitis. It is a miracle she is still alive. Cutting up someone's abdomen is not the treatment for peritonitis. Treatment is washing this abdomen thoroughly and copiously; and where possible, identifying the source of the problem, such as a perforated intestine, perforated appendix or perforated peptic ulcer. I don't know what this guy has. We will search for the usual suspects first," he explained.

"Ba Sir, what is peritonitis?" a porter they called Yikolo asked. He was keenly observing the operation and wondered what peritonitis was.

(Medical Jargon below [*in italics*], may skip without loss to story flow)

"Mr. Yikolo, *Peritonitis is an inflammatory response to peritoneal injury. Injury results in an influx of protein rich fluid, activation of the complement cascade, up-regulation of peritoneal mesothelial cell activity and invasion of the peritoneum with polymorph nuclear neutrophils and macrophages. There is stimulation of cytokine and chemokine production. Bacteria are opsonised and killed by white blood cells and cleared through the lymphatics. The anatomic origin of bacterial contamination and microbiological findings are no major predictors of outcome. However, the preoperative physiological derangement, the surgical clearance of the infectious focus and the response to treatment are established prognostic factors,"* Marx answered smiling at Mr. Yikolo.

"Ba sir, say it in Chimambwe or English please," Mr. Yikolo pleaded with Dr Marx.

"Yikolo, Yikolo, you are just a Porter, don't trouble the doctor, he will just confuse you," one of the people in theatre rebuked the Porter.

"Leave Yikolo alone," Marx answered. "He is a vital member of this treatment team. Never look down on any member of the care team. No matter how humble their job description may appear, it is vital to complete the care chain. If I asked the Matron to empty that suction bottle full of pus over there, she would probably feel insulted. Yet this man Yikolo, he would do it with a smile on his face. Teach him, don't brush him aside."

"Thank you doctor for telling them, these people think my job is not important. I also had wanted to become a doctor when I was young," Yikola answered and went, majestically, to empty the suction bottle that had filled up. Dr Marximillian had just made him feel important.

"My first definition was intended for your doctors. I feel sad none is here to assist in this operation. This was intended to be a platform to exchange and share knowledge and skills. I was sent here for mentorship. I hope it won't turn out to be a vacation for your doctors," said Marx firmly.

"Should I call them?" the coverage asked.

"Leave them, Yikona is here." Marx answered smiling.

"It is Yikolo doctor," the coverage nurse corrected him.

"Very well then, Yikolo; now, peritonitis is inflammation of the peritoneum. The peritoneum is a silk like membrane that lines our inner abdominal wall and covers the organs within our abdomen. Peritonitis is usually due to a bacterial or fungal infection. It can also result from any rupture or perforation in your abdomen, or as a complication of other medical conditions."

Marx showed Yikola the peritoneum in the patient's abdomen and quickly turned his attention to search for the likely causes. He inspected the entire length of small intestines looking for perforations caused by typhoid. He then meticulously examined the appendix; however he found it to be normal by his naked eye inspection. He then directed his search to the stomach to look for perforated ulcers. He found none.

"Fuma fuma konsi kunoli; Konsi kuno fiseme nimakuzana *(Come out come out wherever you are…wherever you are hiding, I am coming to get you)*," he announced in Chimambwe beaming with excitement at the complex surgery he was wrestling with.

He then switched his focus to the Liver. The theatre nurse watched anxiously.

"I didn't know you spoke Mambwe doc," she remarked surprised.

"Good Lord, there you are!" Marx exclaimed when he had found the source of the infection.

"You found it, where was the source of infection?" the Anesthetist asked glad the operation would now come to an end.

"I found a Ghost. I think the gods sent this affliction to test me," Marx announced looking at the anaesthetist. "This boy has empyema of the gall bladder. The entire porta hepatis is inflamed. It is a jungle down there. A Cholecystectomy is unthinkable in our case. This boy is too ill, he was in septic shock. Yikolo, empyema of the Gallbladder or Suppurative Cholecystitis refers to a rare condition in which the Gallbladder is filled with pus. I have never met it in my fourteen years of practice. I have only read about it. This is my first."

"All that smelly pus I emptied in the suction bottle came from his gallbladder," Yikolo answered feeling sorry for the young patient.

"His Gallbladder is perforated. It has a gangrenous patch at its base," Marx spelled out complications he had uncovered.

"What are you going to do doc?" Mr. Njhovu the anaesthetist asked visibly concerned about the turn the operation was likely to take. He worried about the duration the operation might take. It was now, 11pm and he was tired.

"It would be stupid to try to perform a heroic Cholecystectomy in a patient this ill. I will decompress his gall bladder and perform a cholecystostomy instead. Rapture of the gallbladder has a mortality rate of 30%." Marx made his unwavering signature decision. "Yikolo, a cholecystostomy is a procedure where a stoma or mouth or opening is created in the gallbladder, which can facilitate placement of a tube for drainage. It is sometimes used in cases of cholecystitis in which the patient is too ill, and there is a need to delay or defer Cholecystectomy."

Having said this, Marx asked the nurse to pass him a kidney dish. He then proceeded to decompress the gallbladder. It had grown to the size of an adult's gloved fist. Four hundred milliliters of foul smelling pus came oozing out. He then placed a tube inside the gallbladder and secured it. He passed the tube out of the abdomen via another opening on the abdominal wall and attached a collecting bag. Pus could be seen draining immediately. Satisfied with this plumbing he had done, he asked the nurse to prepare the water for washing the interior of the abdomen and all the organs. He washed the patient's abdomen, Liver, spleen, gallbladder, stomach and all the intestines with twelve litres of saline. He was beaming with satisfaction as he did this.

"We are not here to look after fluids; we are here to look after patients. I think hospitals are forgetting their core business nowadays. Every hospital I visit, I find health workers worried about intravenous fluids instead of worrying about their patients. Let us worry about our patients; let he whose job is to supply fluids to the hospitals worry about his job. He is paid for that. Replace him if he is failing in his job. If people should die due to lack of fluids, reflect it in your hospital reports and let the erring officers be punished for negligence of office by public servant. It would be sad to have to write a death certificate; cause of death, No Fluids in the Hospital," he let out a triumphant smirk at his team and scrubbed down.

Dr Marximillian concluded the operation and sent the patient to the ward.

He left Abercorn Community Hospital (ACH) at midnight and headed for his cozy room at Giza. He was tired. Once at the Inn, he took a long hot shower and reflected on Rhoda, a patient inadequately treated for peritonitis. By the time sleep got to him, it was 2am.

**

Home Sweet Home

D r Marximillian woke up at 7. It was a beautiful Monday morning. The sun was shining outside and it was delightfully cool. The weather was set to a perfect 19 degrees centigrade. This would be his first official day at ACH but it didn't feel that way. He had two patients to review that morning. He was deeply concerned about Rhoda and anxious to see Moses, his post Cholecystostomy patient.

He arrived at the hospital and hurried straight to the surgical ward for a ward round. There were several students already on the ward and several other curious faces wanting to see the new guy in their hospital. However, the new guy didn't look new at all. He appeared too free on their wards to be called a visitor. He had an air about him like he owned the ward. He walked around greeting every patient and inspecting the beds and windows in the ward.

"Students, which school are you from?" he asked the students that had come to join him.

"We are General clinical medicine students from Lusaka," one of the students answered.

"Well, what do you call a 'son of a snake'?" Marx asked the students.

They looked at each other confused and searched in vain for the presumed answer he was looking for.

"When I was in first year of medical school, we were taken for community based education to a remote area. We camped at a rural health centre. The next day, a woman was brought to us with a high fever. The community had been told that doctors had come to work at their rural health centre. We told them we couldn't attend to their patient as we were not doctors. Fortunately, a clinical officer came by and saw the patient. When news about this incidence reached the palace of the local headman, he came to see us at once. He had only one question for us. The same question I asked you. And the answer is; the son of a snake is called a snake. The size doesn't matter in snake world. They are all snakes. Similarly, in the eyes of this community and indeed your patients, you are Doctors. Therefore, I shall refer to all of you as Students of Medicine. I don't want to hear this nonsense of *COGs (Clinical Officer General)* students. You are students of medicine from now on and are Doctors in the eyes of the community. Are we clear?" Dr Marximillian gave a short motivational talk to his Medical Students.

"Yes sir," they answered happily.

"Have you seen the post surgery patient?" he asked while walking towards his cholecystostomy patient.

Just then, Dr Kalunda walked into the ward to ask Marx to attend the morning management meeting attended by several community leaders. He was reluctant to be part of this meeting. Nonetheless, he obliged and followed to see what it was they wanted from him. They arrived at the nerve centre of the community hospital. There were several self dignified officials seated on large chairs. The men wore expensive suits and were discussing the affairs of the hospital that had transpired over the weekend. Marx found the night nurse trying to explain why a cholecystostomy had been done at ACH and why so much fluid had been used on just one patient.

"This patient was referred from Mpulungu for intestinal obstruction. An operation was done and appendicectomy, Cholecystectomy....." he fumbled for words as the community leaders stared hard at him.

"Wait, wait, wait; let me help you with that report," said Marx interrupting the night nurse. "This patient had Suppurative Cholecystitis, also referred to as empyema of the gallbladder. He was critically ill as his disease was complicated by perforation of the gallbladder and peritonitis. Owing to this, we performed a cholecystostomy on the patient and peritoneal larvage. He is looking fine this morning. I was doing rounds and was reviewing that patient the night nurse has reported on when you interrupted me to join this meeting."

The community leaders applauded Dr Marximillian and gave him a standing ovation. He wasn't expecting such a thunderous welcome to their humble community hospital. He wasn't quite sure they even understood what he had said.

"The next report is on the fluid position of the hospital; we have only thirty nine litres for the whole hospital. We will try to share these among critical care areas of the hospital," another community leader presented her report.

Marx tried to restrain himself from meddling in the internal affairs of the hospital. However, he decided this was not the best time to remain silent.

"Excuse me Chair, May I comment on your fluid position," he asked for the chairman's approval.

"Yes please do," the chairman answered.

"Thirty nine Litres is a Joke. Fluid shortage such as this ought to be treated as a hospital administrative emergency. Let me put it into perspective for you; one case of peritonitis due to a perforated ulcer or ruptured appendix for that matter would need a minimum of ten litres just for washing the abdomen. Outcome of peritonitis surgery or bowel surgery, especially bowel perforation is directly proportional to how thorough you washed the abdomen. You can perform an excellent operation and repair a perforated intestine or peptic ulcer, but if you neglect to wash that abdomen, chances of your patient dying remain very high. Right now, there is a patient in Gyn ward, named Rhoda. I think most of you may have seen her in the corner of the ward, at the back because she smells too awful to be nursed in the main ward. She was operated on three weeks ago for peritonitis. I reviewed her file yesterday. A brilliant operation was done here at ACH. The only sin that was committed is this; only one litre of Ringer's Lactate was used to wash her abdomen. And is the reason she is still on the ward. Unfortunately she is dying right under our noses. She was inadequately treated. She now has developed what is called tertiary peritonitis. She has also developed severe anaemia. Her Hb is 5g/dl. I plan to operate on her nonetheless. I intend to use twenty litres to clean up the mess your Fluid Rations created. For the time I am here, rest assured, I will finish all your *'tu ma fluids twakupimisha' (your fluid rations)*. Thirty nine litres is a big joke when Mpulungu and the district hospital send all their cases of peritonitis to you."

"That's Dr Marximillian Mukonka Chiti. He has come to help us at our community hospital. I am sure his work is self explanatory from this case he has presented to us. He specializes in very difficult conditions. Dr Marximillian you are welcome to ACH. Make yourself feel at home. You may greet the members present," the chairman introduced Marx to the community leaders.

"Thank you all for inviting me to ACH. I love the weather in your town. I am already enjoying the work. And if you may permit me, I would like to return to my ward to finish my ward round. Enjoy your meeting," he said and rose to leave.

Having ruined the morning meeting for the leaders at ACH, Marx left the command centre located at the basement of the hospital's west wing. He wore a big grin on his face as he strode back to surgical ward.

He found the medical students eagerly waiting for him. A doctor was there too with the students. He was an elderly looking fellow but incredibly humble. Marx immediately liked this fellow.

"Welcome to ACH doctor. I am Dr Mule Nfumu. You can call me Nfumu or Mule. I am in charge of surgical ward," he introduced himself, his face genuinely beaming with Joy.

"I have come to learn from you doc. I guess you have much to show me," Marx replied.

"Not after the case you did last night. You are a great doctor. I have much to learn from you instead. I want you to take over the ward for the time you are here. I'll join my friends here and be a student too," said Dr Nfumu as he moved to the back of the pack.

After this humble transfer of the instruments of surgical power, Dr Marximillian led the team to the bed on which the post Cholecystostomy patient lay.

The team found Moses resting his head on the palm of his right hand. His legs were bent at the knees and rested both his feet on the bed. His hospital blanket was drawn down to his waist. A long white adhesive bandage still covered his surgical wound neatly. A brownish cloudy fluid ran down a tube from the upper aspect of his right abdomen into a collecting bag. His eyes were still deeply jaundiced. An intravenous fluid ran down a line into the veins of his left forearm. Marx's clinical eye was pleased to note the patient's breathing rate had eased down.

"How are you feeling this morning Moses?" he asked the patient.

"Chikuwaya ya docota *(it is paining doctor)*," he answered in Mambwe.

Marx reassured his patient calmly. He then turned to his pack and begun to teach. Several nurses joined the round that morning to take a peek at this mysterious visitor.

(Medical Jargon below [*in italics*], may skip without loss to story flow)

"Cholecystitis occurs most commonly due to blockage of the cystic duct with gallstones. This leads to build up of bile in the gall bladder and increased pressure within the gallbladder, leading to right upper abdominal pain. Concentrated bile, pressure within the gallbladder, and sometimes bacterial infection irritate and damage the gallbladder wall, causing inflammation. This leads to reduced blood flow to areas of the gallbladder and result into cell death. A number of complications may occur from cholecystitis if not detected early or properly treated. Case in point, our patient Moses here," Dr Marximillian explained.

"Is that the reason why pus is coming out of the tube you placed in his gall bladder?" a medical student, O'Neil, asked.

"Why didn't you just remove the gallbladder," another medical student, Esther, asked.

"Dr O'Neil and Dr Esther; urgent decompression is the goal of therapy for empyema of the gallbladder in patients who are hemodynamically unstable or in individuals in whom surgery is contraindicated because of significant comorbid conditions. However, surgical decompression and resection of the affected gallbladder is the criterion standard of therapy. Moses had obscured local Anatomy, high risk of uncontrolled bleeding and there was increased danger to damage nearby structures. This must be born in mind by anyone considering surgical misadventure in this territory of great anatomical variation, especially when working at 23hrs in an Abercorn operating theatre," he explained

Having said this, Dr Marximillian led his pack of young doctors to see Rhoda in Gyn ward. They found Rhoda, now a cast away, attended by a swarm of boorish flies and an offensive reek. Marx's heart sunk when he saw the hemoglobin result. It was dangerously too low. He turned to Dr Nfumu and asked for his opinion.

"There is no blood in the hospital doc, the district hospital has no blood too. She was operated on twice, I don't understand why this disease has not resolved by now, especially given that she has a functioning immune system," he answered.

"Ya docota, ngazwini lolini manzi na mafina yakufuma, yakununka. Mwati ndapola? (Please doctor, help me. Look at this foul smelling fluid and pus coming out. Am I going to recover?)," the patient pleaded with Dr Marximillian to help her.

"We are here to help you honey. Would you allow me to examine you and check where this fluid is coming from?" Marx reassured his patient. However, he did not believe his own words.

While the nurse fetched for a pair of gloves for Marx, the patient lifted her skirt and lay naked in bed. The beddings were she lay were drenched in pus. A horrible odour banged the medical students' olfactory apparatus relentlessly. Marx reached out with his gloved hand and gently slipped it into the patient's vagina. He guided it gently in mire of porridge like fluid, until he reached the cervix and the surrounding areas. He carefully examined the walls of the vagina with his index and middle finger. On the left side of the cervix, an area known as the lateral fornix, Dr Marximillian's hand met no resistance. The hand slid effortless inside till Marx could touch the patient's intestines. The temperature inside was incredibly hot. A deluge of fluid came gushing out when he did this. The reek accompanying this fluid out nearly knocked him over. The patient whimpered and groaned in pain; however she did not close her legs. He then withdrew his gigantic hand and inserted it into the patient's rectum to look for similar communications with the puddle of pus inside her abdomen. When Marx had finished his thorough gynecological assessment, he thanked the patient and turned to his team to teach.

"This patient has tertiary peritonitis. Can anyone tell me why?" Marx asked taking of his gloves. It was past 2pm by now. The students were hungry.

"What is Tertiary peritonitis doctor?" Esther asked.

"Dr Esther, intraperitoneal infection known as peritonitis is a major killer in the practice of clinical surgery. Tertiary Peritonitis, TP, may be defined as intra-abdominal infection that persists or recurs 48 hours following successful and adequate surgical source control," Marx explained to his doctors.

"Are you going to operate on her doctor?" a concerned nurse asked.

"I want to operate on her right now. We need to wash her abdomen thoroughly. At the last operation, her abdomen was washed with only one litre of fluid. This was inadequate treatment and is most likely the reason she developed tertiary peritonitis," he explained.

"Could it be the reason why my post bowel resection patients leak stool and pus one week after operation? I use only one litre of fluid to wash the abdomen. I had to re-operate on several of my patients and unfortunately would be too ill to withstand subsequent surgery," Dr Nfumu asked.

"The key doc is to thoroughly wash the peritoneal cavity. If you don't do it, your patients will develop complications and die from TP," Marx answered. "When theatre can't give you Saline, ask the laboratory to provide you ten litres of distilled water. It will save your patients."

Marx left the hospital late that day with a heavy heart. He couldn't operate on Rhoda as there was no blood in the hospital. He wondered at how many people at ACH were as worried for this patient as he was. He could not sleep that night. He tossed and turned in bed. He tried to forget his patient but her words kept coming at him. *"Ya docota, ngazwini lolini manzi na mafina yakufuma, yakununka; Mwati ndapola? Please doctor, help me....."*

Out of the Heart

Marx awoke the following morning feeling drained. This was his fifth day in Mbala. The sun was shining outside and the weather was a little chilly. His hospital Transport had delayed to pick him. He made himself some coffee and swallowed to cups before the driver arrived. This seemed to have revived him as his mind cleared for the decisions ahead.

On arrival at ACH, Marx rushed straight to the Gyn ward to see Rhoda. He was met by a young doctor who introduced himself as the doctor in charge of Gyn ward. He was a cheerful young fellow and dressed immaculately. Several medical students accompanied this young fellow. He was conducting the ward round when Marx arrived on the ward.

"Dr Marximillian I presume; I am Dr Asum," he introduced himself. "This lady is very ill doctor. I wasn't expecting her to make it to this day."

"Good to meet you. How is she today?" Marx answered getting down to business.

"Her hemoglobin result came back from the laboratory and is very low; 5grams per decilitre. Her vital signs are all deranged and her kidneys are failing," Mr. Mukwisa the nurse on duty answered.

"Life is a mystery my friends. We have no power over life and death. In my short practice, I have attended dying patients that recovered incredibly from their death beds when medically, they should have died. I have learnt to do all I can as a human doctor and to let God do his divine part. I have witnessed many miracles on these hospital beds," said Marx looking at the students.

"I can tell a man by the words of his mouth and by his selfless concern for others. Right now, I can tell you that this doctor is not an ordinary man. The favour of God is upon his life," Dr Asum prophesized to his perplexed students.

"We may receive some blood for Kasama later in the day today. A blood transfusion will help boost her hemoglobin," the nurse explained. She was worried Marx would take the patient to theatre with low hemoglobin.

"It is often very difficult to make decisions over dying people. The temptation to turn away is often very high. We are often convinced their time to die has come and that there is absolutely nothing that can be done to help them. Patients are abandoned to die, even those we could have done something about and added a day to their life. Personally, I would rather kill you trying to help you than sit and watch you die," Marx explained to his perplexed audience.

"But how would you know what God wants you to do," Jessica asked with a puzzled look on her youthful face.

"Dr Jessica, personally, I try not to think what God thinks. Remember his ways are not our ways and his thoughts are as high as the heavens are from earth. To put it in Astrophysics language, his thoughts and ways are an infinite light years from ours," said Marx.

"So we shouldn't even try to think like God. We should just stick to our human thoughts and job descriptions; is it not written that when someone is taken ill, he must call on the elders of the church to pray for him," said Johnny scratching his long beard.

"Those who are quick to conclude at outcomes of events in the world, including death; alleging that it was the will of God, such and such happened; often times speak on behalf of gods they carry in their pockets," Marx explained further.

"Most speak out of ignorance," Jessica agreed.

"They are often times liars, cheats and hypocrites," said Johnny.

"Who appointed them to speak his mind on the likely outcome of desperately sick people?" Dr Asum asked.

"Our job is solely to render our hand at our patient's dire circumstance. Personally, I make human decisions. Years ago, I asked God to allow me to think as a man that I am. Never as a god for that is not what I am. However, I also asked him to help me recognize his often tranquil still voice. I am a man of flesh and blood and anything that my abilities and training can do, I will do. I find famers to be the most fascinating people on earth. They never go to a piece of forest chanting and expecting God to come down to plough their forest and plant seed for them," Marx explained leaning on a hospital bed.

"This is not to say we must not pray; God said, 'I am the Lord your Healer.' learn when to sow and when to reap, when to stand and when to sit, when to walk and when to stop. God can use anyone. He can even use a stone to care for a patient. He is no respecter of persons," Dr Asum preached.

All the patients and their relatives on the ward were profoundly astonished at what they were hearing their doctors discuss. They wondered at what manner of a doctor this was and his team. The ward had become a place of worship. Everyone was quiet except for babies in the adjacent pediatric ward and a maid's vacuum cleaner in the corridor leading to Maternity ward. Many patients had never seen doctors who believed in God.

"You know doc, last week during my night call, I was called to review Rhoda on this same bed. The nurse told me she had changed condition. When I arrived on the ward, I found truly so she had. She was gasping for air. I was sure she would not live to see the next morning. There was nothing else left to do as the nurse had already commenced the patient on oxygen and some intravenous fluids. I made a diagnosis of Systemic inflammatory response syndrome (SIRS). She already had been through two operations to treat the cause. The only thing I was left to do doc, was to take off my outer coat and put on my inner coat. I went to the side ward, knelt down and earnestly prayed for Rhoda," Dr Asum revealed his pious inner self.

"I do not understand SIRS, please explain it to us," Joan, an incredibly pretty Brazilian medical student said looking at Marx.

"I love your dreadlocks Dr Joan. How long have you been growing it?" Marx asked.

"Thank you Sir," she answered. "I've had it for four years now."

"SIRS is the body's response to an infectious or non infectious insult. Although the definition of SIRS refers to it as an inflammatory response, it actually has pro- and anti- inflammatory components. As of this year 2016 however, SIRS was completely eliminated from the definition of sepsis. The complications of SIRS include; Acute lung injury, Shock, multiple organ dysfunction syndrome and Acute kidney injury," Dr Marximillian explained smiling at Joan.

He liked this amazing student doctor, only she didn't know it. He would look out for her from that day onwards.

"Mr. Mukwisa lets prepare Rhoda for laparotomy. Inform theatre about her and obtain consent. I don't know why God has chosen to use surgery to cure this lady. You kept her here to wait for me. I had difficulties sleeping last night. I kept thinking about Rhoda," Marx announced decisively. "Dr Jessica and Dr Joan you are scrubbing in with me."

***

The anaesthetist was visibly sad when he saw Rhoda in theatre that morning. He was not prepared to accept this patient without a fight. Marx was no stranger to operating theatre battles. He beat the anesthetists easily and squarely on many similar battles. He was fully prepared for the battle that awaited him in theatre that morning. He decided he would first play hide and seek with the anaesthetist in this colossal theatre. In so doing, Marx hoped reality would sink in the mind of the anaesthetist. When he finally caught up with Marx in the boiler room, he laid his arguments with naked displeasure. The boiler room was located in the inner ring of this gigantic theatre complex.

"Doc, why are you bringing this patient with low hemoglobin to theatre?" he argued.

"Because I want to exorcise the demon eating her hemoglobin," he answered.

"She will die. She won't be able to survive surgery and anesthesia. She is too ill to survive. Couldn't you wait for blood?" He continued visibly angry.

"She will only grow weaker. Look at what waiting has brought her; I think it is immoral to let another day pass while we stand and do nothing," Marx answered firmly.

They were joined by the theatre nurse who had gone to check on the voices coming out of the boiler room as it was not far from the store room. She had gone there to pick sutures and fluids.

"Last time I scrubbed on this same patient, the abdomen was completely frozen. We couldn't even reach her Uterus. We couldn't examine her intestines; they were all stuck together. We had a visiting surgeon just like you have come," the theatre nurse warned Dr Marximillian and spelt out the difficult operation she witnessed on Rhoda.

"Don't worry about what you found, we may find worse," Marx retorted. "Just go ahead and prepare your table. I will have two assistants."

The anaesthetist left with the nurse mumbling to each other.

"Should I prepare a major lap set?" she called out from the wide passage leading to the recovery room.

"Prepare for the worst case scenario," he answered smiling to himself.

Marx was aware; it needn't have to be that way. They were all concerned about the same patient. However, Marx was not prepared to leave his patient at the mercy of SIRS and Sepsis. He wanted to thoroughly wash out the pus in Rhoda's abdomen, the source of her infection.

***

Rhoda was laid on the operating table at 2pm. Jessica and Joan walked into theatre looking incredibly beautiful. Joan wore tight blue scrubs that greatly accentuated her amazing female persona. She was a marvel to behold. Her eyes sparkled like a pair of diamonds in the slit left by her mask and cape. Her hips angled benevolently in her blue trousers. Jessica stood by her side looking stunning herself. They were like a pair of beautiful identical twins. Theatre Scrubs had power to increase a lady's beauty exponentially.

"You look extremely beautiful girls," the anaesthetist remarked looking at the girls. His face had brightened up for the first time since coming into theatre that afternoon.

The girls giggled and smiled behind their blue masks. Marx walked in and greeted the girls candidly.

"Ladies, you look stunning. Are you ready for the party? Come, let us scrub in," he said leading the way to the spacious scrubbing station.

The nurse was waiting for them on her instrument table. As soon as she had gowned the surgeons, Marx led the team into the operating room. He proceeded to clean the patient's abdomen and covered her in a green sheet. A large circular light, hovered above and shone brightly on the patient's abdomen. Marx approached the operation table and re examined the abdomen through a wide window in the drape

After a brief moment, he re-opened the patient's abdomen via her old scar. The wound was still fresh and its edges easily gave way to light pressure. Pus came oozing out as soon as he entered the abdomen.

Joan stood on his right. Her body was radiating intense heat standing close to Marx like that. A phenomenon Marx called *MOSS* and greatly appreciated however made no mention about it. Fuelled by his androgens, he grinned and let his mind wander away. He was completely enveloped by Joan's heat signature. Theatre was cold that afternoon. Jessica and the theatre nurse stood across the table unaware of the chemistry Joan's body had ignited. Marx was on fire.

"I didn't know it was this easy to enter a recently operated abdomen," Jessica remarked.

"Did you see, he simply tore through it," the theatre nurse observed.

Joan drew away from Marx. He noticed and smiled, "Dr Joan, you needn't be scared of me. Just move close to me. Don't be scared."

"Move close to the doctor till you are rubbing against each other. This is theatre my dear, that's the only way if you are to see clearly what he is doing," the theatre nurse encouraged Joan.

"I was afraid I would disturb him," she answered naively. Everyone burst out laughing at her.

"Don't worry about him. He actually needs that," the anaesthetist remarked. There was more laughter in theatre.

He was pleased seeing the patient was not bleeding at all.

Marx gently moved his hand over the matted intestines. He managed to separate all loops of bowels. Then he directed his attention to look for the uterus, which he found easily. It was normal in appearance together with its fallopian tubes. Further down, in an area where large arteries exited the abdominal cavity, he found a large tunnel communicating with the vagina outside. This tunnel had been burrowed by the stream of pus trying to exit the body alongside the blood vessels. This passage was the reason for the continuous leak of foul smelling fluid Rhoda had complained about to Marx. The burrow extended deep below at the back to reach the left kidney. Marx picked Joan's hand and gently guided it to feel the gaping crater inside their patient's abdomen.

"Oh my God, it is so big," Joan exclaimed.

"What's so big?" the Anaesthetist asked with a grin on his face. "This is theatre Dr Joan; you would be surprised what people listening through the window would think you were referring to."

There was more laughter in theatre when the anesthetist made this insinuating remark.

"Let me feel it too," Jessica asked.

"Leave the young girls alone Mr. Mema," said Dr Asum. He had just walked into theatre.

"Why weren't we able to do this in her first operation?" the theatre nurse asked perplexed. "I was on the operation table myself and I recall the intestines were firmly adhered inside her abdomen. We couldn't even see her uterus."

"It is the Inner Coat sister," Jessica answered smiling.

The operation lasted only twenty minutes. Marx and the girls washed Rhoda's intestines thoroughly till only clear fluid was coming out of the abdomen. They placed a drain on the left side of her abdomen. They placed a second drain through the burrow they had discovered inside the abdomen leading to the left lateral fornix; the opening Marx had felt when he had examined Rhoda on the ward.

***

A Wild Goose Chase

S tubborn thoughts of disappointment weighed heavily on his surgical mind as he left theatre at 4 pm. He was hungry and tired. His patient, Rhoda was sent to the ward for critical care nursing.

His request for a bailout had been turned down by *The System*. He was bankrupt. His only source of income, his meager salary had been blocked by *The System*, following a court order to divert his salary to his adorable ex-wife, a *Chez Ntemba She-Devil*.

Marx was beginning to feel the actions taken against him take a toll. He was struggling not to cry. He couldn't buy a snack in town or take the girls that had assisted in Rhoda's surgery for a drink on the shores of Lake Chila. He walked slowly to his lodge wondering whether anyone cared anything at all. He was on the verge of tipping into self pity. However, he chose to laugh at his own misery.

He had the sense to know, he was not indispensable. He knew a human resource scout would not shilly-shally to give out his position if it fell vacant. They would simply fill it with anything on two legs, even four legs. He was sure; the cartel did not feel for devout workers like him. None was attached to the people they served as Marx was to his patients. He was merely a position in the ruthless scheme run by the Position Filling Scouts. In Marx's mind, it couldn't be called a Human Resource development because it lacked a conscience. If he left, Cockroaches, Jackals, Monkey and Rats could be recruited to take his position and set loose to slay millions. Provided positions were filled, the Positions filling Cartel couldn't care less.

He was certain the Cartel had failed to diagnose the dire state of his basic livelihood. He had been falsely accused and his name scandalized. For how could a man passionately devoted to his patients; the poor and disadvantaged, sick strangers, women and children, be accused of child abandonment?

The decision taken by the court to give his salary away to a whore and *The System's* decision to deny him a bailout plan was beginning to seem like a conspiracy against him. Marx was certain his life was under siege. He had tried calling on the heavens to intervene in his predicament, but for some unclear reasons, his God too had gone silent on him. Marx had never felt as alone in the world as he did on that cold Mbala afternoon.

He reflected on Daliso's five year debt siege in a rural school and countless other frustrated teachers saving at various schools country wide. For the first time, Marx saw somber resemblance in his work and that for several teachers. It suddenly dawned on him; a frustrated human resource could be a grave danger to the community as well as to the System, when they chose to vent their frustration and unleash personal vendetta on the people they were expected to serve.

***

Marx sat in his room at Giza Inn struggling to resist the forces of evil trying to turn him into a cruel cold hearted assassin. He reflected on how he ended up in that miserable profession as a doctor.

Marx had been a bright kid at school. He loved working with people greatly. However, as a high school pupil, he hated hospitals and school laboratories. His mother thought he would make a fine doctor even though he hated the smell of medicines in hospitals and chemicals in chemistry laboratories.

The long odious study to becoming a doctor offered his bright mind great appeal to conquer all examinations that lay on the way to graduation day. Marx loved exams deeply and enjoyed preparing for them. His natural ability to work with his hands naturally guided him into surgery. Money had never crossed his mind as a factor for the work he did. His greatest reward had always been the joy of seeing his patients rise from their sick beds and walk home. Provided he had just enough food to give him strength for one day at a time, he would go on working to care for the sick that came to seek his knowledge and skill.

Unfortunately, the order of his world and philosophy was being threatened by the cruel treatment he was receiving. It now appeared to him; it was all about the money. Just as a live dog was worth more than a dead Lion, it was now clear to Marx, a dead Chihuahua could be worth more than a bankrupt doctor.

Marx reflected on his trip to Mbala; he was sure, if it was worth anything at that moment; it was his encounter with Rhoda and Moses.

Later that night at 8pm, he decided to make a call to *The System's* Finance Manager to find out why his request for a bailout had been declined. He called several times, but the phone went unanswered. Marx had known for a long time; mobile phones went largely unanswered for several reasons, including; the caller's call being deemed inappropriate, the caller presumed to be asking for money or the caller considered a social nuisance by the person being called. Dr Marximillian had made the social nuisance category of this officer's call list.

When he finally got to Marx, he spoke with impunity and disrespected a senior officer.

"You are over sixty percent in debt doctor. The committee couldn't approve your request for a salary advance owing to your careless debt. You are what we call a high risk employee to lend money to," Mr. Munalula answered.

"Don't you people have financial grants to bail out employees like me," he asked.

"We can't help you mister, just try to find another way to reduce your debt burden. Didn't you get yourself into this?" Munalula replied.

Marx thought for a moment and cut the line. The pain of tears building up under his eye lids blinded him momentarily. He was on the verge of crying.

He deeply regretted the glitter of hope the prospects of a bailout plan had brought him. It was his biggest mistake yet chasing *The System* for help. He had waited for two months only to get this rebuff to his face. He prayed neither this fellow nor his relatives would trespass to Marx's theatre in their life time.

Marx, knew when these fellows needed help they could call till they killed someone's phone battery. Those they called would not have peace of mind while the phone rang.

He recalled a distress call he once received from a politician who had tried to frustrate him at work. Mr. Silly Moyo had served in a government that had since been booted out of power. He had called Dr Marximillian frantically one Sunday evening when his brother was suddenly taken ill and later admitted for intestinal obstruction. Marx was not the only doctor at the hospital. Mr. Silly's patient could be attended to by anyone. Unfortunately that anyone erred in his diagnosis, nearly ending in a fatality. Marx was what you would call a few good doctors.

When Silly's relative was suddenly taken ill, he was referred from a district hospital, 300km from Marx's hospital. Being a good man he was, Marx operated on Mr. Silly's brother and saved his life even when he was not the one on duty in theatre that Sunday evening.

Dr Marximillian was lured into debt by a small business he was courting. His startup company crashed leaving him wallowing in debt. When he was about to get up, his misery was followed by a cold blooded court case which ended with his salary being taken away. He was aware this money was not going towards the welfare of his lovely children; instead, it was being channelled to fund the bottomless whoring pit of Satan. A hole now patronized by many that were hounding him. A restless void that could not be filled by all their disgusting bodily fluids discharged into its Abyss.

Several covert operatives knew all the fornicators and adulterers that had slandered Marx's name to his beautiful ex wife, a poisoned chalice. It was only by defaming Marx they could relieve their disgusting bodily waste into the restless whoring pit of Satan. She took great pleasure at being pitied and sold her body to anything pretending to lend its ear. She listened to their disgusting slanderous tongues about the Honorable Dr Marximillian with devilish fascination and intent.

Marx's former patients, working as clandestine operatives, believed Marx was a good man. Otherwise no one would give a damn talking in derogatory terms about him. Marx knew the devil did not waste time with pimps, midgets and punks. He fought moral men, good men, noble people, a few good doctors; men and women destined for great works.

Satan will fight anyone called to serve God's people. As far as Marx was concerned, the real crime he had committed was to stand up and offer himself to the service of God's people. The devil was determined to extinguish the gift God had bestowed upon his life.

Marx had an incredible gift that allowed him to see into many patients' illnesses. He could transmit God's healing to the critically ill by the skill of his hand. However he hadn't fully comprehended how his hands worked. He still had much to learn and mature. He was still raw and wild at heart.

***

Marx stayed up late that night nursing a terrible headache. At that hour, he despised the Hippocratic Oath in its entirety. Nevertheless, he would always be overwhelmed and remain in awe of it.

Often, he was gripped by a deluge of nostalgic memories, how as a young doctor he had sworn to be bound by it, to do no harm. Beaming with pride, he and his Graduand Comrades, dubbed the millennium medics, had sworn by various Greek healing gods to uphold specific ethical tenets of historical and traditional value. He recited the oath to himself in his cold room at the Inn;

"I Swear by Apollo the physician and Asclepius,
by Hygeia and Panacea and by all the gods and goddesses
as my witnesses that I will carry out,
according to my ability
and judgment, this oath and this contract.
To hold my teacher in this Art equal to my own parents
to make him partner in my livelihood;
when he is in need of money to share mine with him;
to consider his family as my own brothers,
and teach them this art, if they want to learn it,
without fee or contract;
to impart precept, oral instruction,
and all other instruction to my own sons,
the sons of my teacher,
and to indentured pupils who have taken the physician's oath,
but to nobody else…."

That night, Marx was convinced he had made the biggest mistake of his life, swearing by those inanimate Greek gods. He recalled an oath by a chongololo monk, a student from D block, a notorious hostel for medical students at the medical school he attended;

"I swear this shit is all about the money,

I swear to go forth from this day forward

and make me some dole

by whatever means possible

I swear, I shall refuse to be used cheaply,

Everyone consulting must pay

or let them fry

this shit is all about the f**kn Money doc."

Marx was certain Hippocrates himself would have been horrified at the modified oath that still bears his name. Where he had said;

"I will use those dietary regimens which will benefit
my patients
according to my greatest ability and judgment,
and
I will do no harm or injustice to them.
I will not give a lethal drug to anyone if I am asked,
nor will I advise such a plan;
and similarly
I will NOT give a woman
a pessary to cause an abortion "

Doctors had long wandered away; they had invented their own convenient miniature oaths. Apollo, Asclepius and Hygeia, including their faithful servant Hippocrates would be horrified at the millions of unborn babies being slain by pessaries administered to women and girls. It was now clear to Marx; it was all about the money. He was almost certain, the chongololo monk had been right; it is all about the money.

At midnight, he suddenly found himself missing Ms Isaacs, the girl who bent the fabric of time, turning his crawling bus into a Great North Maglev. However, he dared not call her. He was sure she had already looked him up on the credit reference bureau listing for individuals wallowing in debt. She was too smart to waste her time on a Castrated Mbala Bull. She was too busy chasing wild Chihuahuas online to think of a fisherman she met on a midnight bus trip.

***

It was business as usual at the Hospital the next day. It was Friday, Marx's seventh day in Mbala. He spent the morning conducting rounds on the wards. Moses was looking great that morning. He was eating his regular diet. Pus from his gall bladder tube had been replaced by a green liquid which Dr Marximillian called bile. Moses' eyes had cleared out. He looked ready to going home, however Marx decided to keep him till the following week.

He discharged other patients he had operated on since arriving in Mbala. There was a boy, aged thirteen, on the first bed on the right just after the acute bay looking anxiously at him. Three days earlier, Marx removed a chest tube Dr Nfumu had inserted in the boys right chest following a near fatal fall that left his left chest fill up with blood and air; a condition Dr Nfumu called heamopneumothorax.

"uli uli, (*how are you*)," Marx greeted the anxious boy.

"Nile Ningo ya docota (I am fine doctor)," the boy answered with a shy smile.

Marx checked the boy's chest and after being satisfied with his air entry, he certified him fit to go home. The boy jumped from his bed excitedly. He dashed across to a bed by the window where another thirteen year old waited anxiously to be seen.

"Ukunvwa uli (*how are you feeling*)" Marx asked the second boy while his friend looked on.

"Chikuwaya sile panono (it is paining just a little)," the boy answered looking down.

"Ukulonda kuya ku ng'anda (*would you like to go home*)," he asked.

"Nkulonda (*I would like to go*)," he answered visibly delighted and turned to his friend excitedly.

"Yawen ya kwiza mukuku senda (*who is coming to get you*)," Marx asked.

"Ya Tate (*my father*)," he replied and staggered out of the bed excitedly in the company of his newly found friend.

The two boys ran around the ward visibly thrilled. They bade farewell to people they had met while on the ward. They went over to Moses' bed and bade him farewell. These two boys had met on the ward and quickly developed a strong bond. At ACH, children and adults shared the same ward. Marx castrated the second boy three days earlier. Each testis weighed over a kilo at surgery and made walking an extreme ordeal for this boy. Marx was sure, this boy had testicular cancer. Unfortunately, access to pathology services did not exist at the hospital. Samples had to be sent over one thousand kilometres away and took years for results to return.

"Dr Marximillian, does it mean Mike will never have children of his own when he grows up?" Jessica asked visibly concerned for Mike.

"I am afraid so my dear," he answered walking out of surgical ward.

Marx left the ward with Jessica. He wanted to see Rhoda in Gyn ward. She was now day one post surgery. He was hoping blood for transfusion had come from Kasama. The other students remained behind to write discharge certificates and prescriptions. They discussed Mike among themselves.

"He said the boy had testicular cancer. I wonder why he chose to castrate him instead of taking just a small piece. He could have spared his balls?" Shifu spoke in his heavy croaky voice.

"At least he can walk without that heavy weight pulling of his scrotum. I weighed those testes in theatre. They had a combined total weight of two and half kilos," Ethel told his friends

"I wonder how he managed to get around with all that weight. I didn't know, you guys your balls could grow to this size. Not even a bull's issues grow to that size," Selym remarked looking at Shifu and Johnny.

"Do you want to examine us?" Johnny asked with a grin on his face.

"Jump on the bed," Selym answered pointing to an empty bed on the right.

"Let's follow Dr Marximillian; he has gone to see Rhoda. Joan, ask him to tell us the likely cancer that did this to this poor boy," Shifu told his friends.

"Why don't you ask him yourself?" Joan answered.

"You can't see that he likes you. I think you like him too. In theatre he only asks you to assist him. He makes us feel left out," Johnny complained.

"That's why I don't come to theatre," said Fred.

"I can't believe you guys are jealous. How can you think such things? Dr Marx loves everyone. Thoughts like that will just cost you an opportunity to learn. Mind you, we are here for school and are privileged to have a very good Teacher visiting ACH," Joan answered laughing.

***

Meanwhile on Gyn ward, Marx and Jessica found Rhoda fully awake. She was visibly happy to see Dr Marximillian. The smell that had habited her bed left her. She was combing her hair while her husband fed her an orange. Unfortunately she had not yet received blood. She was deeply anaemic. The other students had caught up and stood around their teacher eager to learn.

"Dr Marximillian, that boy in male surgical ward; what cancers would grow that fast? His parents told us he has just been unwell for seven weeks," Shifu asked and winked at Joan.

(Medical Jargon below [*in italics*], may skip without loss to story flow)

"Leukaemia and Lymphoma are the most common secondary malignancies to affect the testes. These tumors can present bilaterally as

was the case with Mike, and, because the Blood-Testis barrier protects the intratesticular cells, the testis may be the site of residual tumor in children after chemotherapy. Metastatic disease to the testes should be considered in a child presenting with bilateral testicular tumors. Paratesticular structures can give rise to various benign conditions such as; lipoma, Leiomyoma, hemangioma, fibroma, etc and malignant tumors; however these are extremely rare. Rhabdomyosarcoma is the most common malignant tumor. It may arise from the distal spermatic cord and appear as a scrotal mass or hydrocele. These tumors have a bimodal distribution and occur in boys aged 3-4 months and in Teenagers. Up to 70% of cases involve the retroperitoneal lymph nodes at presentation," Dr Marximillian spelled out the differential diagnoses in their patient.

"Is Mike going to be ok?" Joan asked visibly concerned.

"These tumors are highly aggressive my dear," Marx answered resting his big left hand tenderly on Joan's left shoulder. "*They spread via the blood, lymphatics, or direct extension to lungs, the cortical bone, or to the bone marrow in 20% of patients at the time of diagnosis. Radical inguinal orchiectomy, followed by retroperitoneal lymph node dissection is recommended for all children older than 10 years.*

I am impressed with all your concerns. It is the first step to joining the league of a few good doctors. Let us talk about Rhoda now."

***

Marx left the Hospital at 2pm. He strolled into town along President Avenue where he was surprised to find a heavy presence of police in riot gear. Some wore combat regalia. He walked towards the war memorial round about. A convey of police cars passed him and some officers sneered at pedestrians. The people simply went about their business. No one paid any special attention at this police circus in town.

There was a rumour a leading opposition political leader would be visiting town. The police had been set loose to thwart his plans to meet the local people. They were deployed to gun down freedom of speech. It was clear to Marx; the local people could not be fooled any more. He found the locals to be extremely wonderful people. They had no time for megalomaniacs. The era for pathological egotists had no room in Mbala.

Only people with delusions of grandeur and an obsession with power would go to such lengths and brandish assault rifles, machine guns and tanks at a peaceful citizenry. Marx didn't need to be a political scientist to read the political landscape in Mbala. All the people Marx engaged on the subject greatly admired the American political league playing out during that same period. Had Mbala been a US state, Marx was certain the whole town would have turned out in large numbers to hear Hillary and Bernie Sanders speak. They would even have heard out Ted Cruz, Donald Trump, John Kirsch, Jeb Bush and Ben Carson.

While this political league was playing out in America, Leicester, a Thai owned club was on course to win their first ever historical English premier league Title. A very unlikely football fairy tale in the English Premier League history was about to be become legend at birth. Everyone in the small town of Mbala was too busy watching this fairy tale play out to waste their precious time on a clown army loitering in their beautiful town.

Marx strode down President Avenue after the police had driven out. He passed the junction to Mbala secondary school and walked leisurely down admiring the gorgeous pine trees lining the road. He met two young men on a bicycle near the 'Slope', a small leisure spot on the road side. They were discussing politics.

"*Starsky* and *Hutch* are at my uncle's farm. They arrived last night," the young man pushing the bicycle told his friend.

"Really; Are they here in Mbala?" his friend asked excitedly.

"These two are unstoppable. They are winning this year. I am going to the farm to see them," the two young men talked, walking towards town.

It was deeply regrettable; Africa was still grappling with politics of intimidation, police brutality, suppression of the freedom of speech and association in the 21st century.

***

Marx returned to his room at Giza Inn thinking about buffoons he had met in town. By now it was 6 pm. He was very hungry. He hadn't had lunch. He wanted to eat nothing but Tanganyika breams. When he got to the restaurant, he found it closed. He later learnt that the owners of this wonderful Inn were devout seventh day Adventists. They had closed the restaurant to welcome the Sabbath and would remain closed till Sunday morning. Marx nearly dropped dead when he received this sad news.

He reached his room and begun to search his bags for biscuits. Marx always kept biscuits in his traveling bag as an emergency food source. He was very glad when he found his scrumptious stock still intact.

***

After his biscuit meal, he lay in bed watching television. The news was riddled with global human crisis of immense proportion; earth quakes, floods, financial crisis, famine and war. Marx was certain his own predicaments could make a news item.

Europe was still grappling with the Refugee crisis. Many nations were erecting fences to prevent emigrants from entering their countries. Millions of people had been displaced from their home lands by war. Unfortunately, many European nations had forgotten the pains of war. Only one leader had opened her borders to the suffering refugees. The Angel of Europe, Ms Angela Merkel, welcomed the strangers in their millions.

Everyone else had forgotten the suffering the Second World War and more recently the Balkan war had brought on their nations and the mass human exodus it ushered. Marx listed the notorious Balkan states in his mind; Bosnia and Herzegovina, Kosovo, Slovenia, Croatia, Serbia, Montenegro, Romania, Bulgaria, Albania, Greece, Macedonia and the European part of Turkey. Majority of these states were xenophobic or synonymous with genocide and civil war in his mind. Marx had been in high school when the Bosnian war made headlines in the news and displaced a multitude from their homes. Since then, he had never heard of anything good come out of Bosnia or other Balkan states except for Croatia which had some great football talents. It seemed as though Lucifer's HQ was located in the Balkan before he moved it to Syria.

The Bosnian war was an international armed conflict that took place in Bosnia and Herzegovina between 1992 and 1995. The main belligerents were the forces of the republic of Bosnia and Herzegovina and those of the self-proclaimed Bosnian Serb and Bosnian Croat entities within Bosnia and Herzegovina, Republika Srpska and Herzeg-Bosnia, who were led and supplied by Serbia and Croatia respectively. This war was part of the breakup of Yugoslavia. Following the Slovenian and Croatian secessions from the Socialist Federal Republic of Yugoslavia in 1991; the Serbian government of Slobodan Milosevic and others, mobilized their forces to secure Serb territory. The war soon spread across the country accompanied by ethnic cleansing of the Bosniak and Croat population, especially in eastern Bosnia and throughout the Republika Srpska.

As for the Second World War, many Europeans fled their homes and migrated to North and South America, including Australia. Their hosts were very kind to them unlike this cruel European crop Marx was watching; it was too young and naïve to comprehend the mass human exodus playing out in the media. For many in Europe this was merely a Holy Wood war movie and for left wing politicians, a stage to gain political mileage.

The Libyan, Iraq and Syrian wars and were yet another despicable scourge on human history. It was these wars that had unleashed a deluge of refugees Europe was grappling with, including Daesh. World leaders appeared to have done little to end the hostilities.

The United States' Secretary of State, John Kelly, had done all he could to end the violence. The war was taking a huge toll on him despite being a decorated military man himself. Marx could not remember the last time he saw secretary Kelly smile. He tried to imagine a world governed by Putin and Trump. It would be the end of the world. Unfortunately, the forces controlling a new world order were working tirelessly to unleash unimaginable Mayhem and rile even Putin, Daesh, Assad and Kim Jong-Un.

The evil reincarnates of Lucifer's embodiments on earth, Saddam Hussein, Gaddafi, Bin Laden, Ahmadinejad and Hitler, where enjoying the winds blowing across the Americas. Marx was convinced this was just a tip of the ice berg; dangerous times were lurking ahead, on street corners in every city in the world. Evil men and women, possessed by Lucifer were everywhere, cold blooded murderers, blandishing guns and bombs strapped to their bodies; ready to explode them and slay millions. Marx knew it wouldn't be long before these demoniacs lay their hands on nuclear weapons. These were Satan's newest war generals sworn to unleash havoc on peaceful citizens of the earth. They came out of demon holes in great numbers and changed the rules of war.

While Marx grappled with the turmoil in the world and his own life, his phone rang. He was urgently wanted at the hospital. He looked at his watch, the hour hand pointed harshly to 10pm. He knew this would be a long night. The biscuits he had munched rapidly vaporized from his gut. Suddenly he began to feel very hungry once again. He reached out for a biscuit and placed his cell phone against his ear. It was the coverage night nurse speaking.

"Dr Asum said we could call you. We have received an emergency," the nurse spoke with audible tachycardia over the phone.

"Where is Asum?" Marx asked. His recent persecutions had sucked out every passion for work from his bones. For the first time in his life, he found it hard to respond to an emergency with enthusiasm.

"He is not around sir," the nurse answered. "Can I send a vehicle to pick you?"

Dr Marximillian was suffering from Burnout; a type of psychological stress characterized by exhaustion, lack of enthusiasm and motivation, feeling of ineffectiveness, and also may have the dimension of frustration or cynicism, and as a result reduced efficacy within the workplace.

Marx reluctantly agreed to be picked at the Inn. It was very cold outside. A full moon in the night sky looked down disapprovingly at him. The Milky Way Galaxy appeared unusually too close to earth. Billions of stars shone brightly in the sky. Marx wished he had been an astronaut. He hated his job greatly at that hour. He was starving despite working day and night. Foolish myopic midgets had taken away his salary. He was sure, this was the pain Daliso may have experienced each time he stood in front of his young learners, whom he called his class.

He arrived at the hospital and rushed to Labour ward. He found his patient had already been wheeled into theatre. He passed through a passage connecting labour ward and the operating theatre. This passage opened into a recovery room. There were six beds in the recovery room. He changed shoes at a red line marking the sterility transition zone. He crossed the red line and entered into the ACH theatre complex. Marx greatly loved this grand theatre.

He found the patient already place on the operating table. The anaesthetist was busy giving his equipment a final thorough check. In the next room, the theatre nurse was setting her instruments table. This would be Marx's first caesarean section in Mbala. The nurse was nervous as she didn't know what to expect from the new surgeon. She was an elderly lady who had given 35 years of her life to the operating theatre. She was at ACH as a volunteer. She had never met Marx.

Jessica and Joan had come to theatre to assist Dr Marximillian. They looked pretty in their scrubs as always. Marx was pleased to see the girls. They boosted his fading morale. He thought the girls looked sexy in their blue scrubs. Joan's scrubs hugged her feminine legs tightly and clearly magnified her feminine gluteal and groin anatomical crevices.

"You look beautiful guys," he told the girls.

"Thank you," Joan answered shifting her weight from one leg to the other.

"Where are the others? How many are you in Obstetrics?" he asked.

"We told them. We are six," Jessica answered.

"I sent them back doctor. We have run out of scrubs. These two have their own scrubs," the theatre nurse answered in the next room.

"Are you ready? Can I scrub?" he asked.

"Yes doctor," she answered.

"What is the normal duration of a caesarean section in this theatre," he asked.

"It is one hour doctor," she answered.

"Prepare for two hours then. I will have an assistant," he said. "Joan you will assist me."

"Two hours doctors, you will kill us. It is late. Can we call a doctor to assist? Dr Amber is the fastest here. His Caesars last only thirty minutes sometimes," the anaesthetist protested.

"There is no any other doctor around. They have all gone to Lusaka. It is only Dr Marximillian left in Mbala," the night coverage nurse answered.

There was a sudden silence in theatre. Everyone was sad at the prospects of being taken hostage in theatre for two hours with a slow surgeon. Marx was certain they were cursing him in their hearts. He had not disclosed to them his caesarean exploits elsewhere. The team in theatre was unaware, a record was about to be set in their theatre for the quickest caesarean section performed in Mbala. Marx had set many records in several theatres across the country but chose to keep quiet about these. He had the moral conscience not to turn caesarean births into a sport and pursuit for record breaking titles.

He approached the operating table calmly. He looked at Joan across the table. He winked at her when their eyes met. She knew Marx had a secret hidden under his sleeve.

"Knife please," he said looking at the theatre nurse. "And permission to start."

"The patient is ready," the anesthetist answered impatiently.

"The midwife, you may want to hold the baby receiving towel in your hands right now and I hope your resuscitation table is ready," said Marx smiling at the midwife.

"I will when you reach the uterus doctor," she answered.

"I am afraid you won't see any of that," he answered. "Please turn off the suction machine, it is making noise. I rarely use it for my Caesareans."

Having said this, he picked the knife and made an incision extending down to rectus sheath. He turned the knife in his had and using his index finger he dissected the loose tissues and peritoneum and reached the uterus in the twinkling of an eye. He flipped his surgical knife forwards again and made an elliptical incision at the front of the uterus, in an area known as the lower segment.

"I call this smiling face incision," he announced looking at his hypnotized team.

He put the knife down, and delivered a female baby in a pool of porridge like foul smelling material, which he called meconium grade four. He did all this in just twenty seconds. The midwife woke up from her hypnotic state and fumbled for a receiving towel. Marx cut the cord and passed the baby to Joan as the midwife was not ready.

"He warned you to be ready. Look at you now," the anesthetist remarked at the nurse.

"Please help me with the resuscitation station," she begged the anesthetist still shocked by the speed of the operation.

Marx had delivered the placenta by now and was closing the uterine wound. The theatre nurse had never seen anything like this in all her thirty five years of work. The Caesar was over within seven minutes from the starting time.

"Alimwi inga waseka. Chilagambya echi (*you can end up laughing, this is truly amazing*)," remarked the theatre nurse in her mother tongue.

Marx left Joan on the operating table to dress the wound. He walked to the scrub station to wash his hands and change his theatre shoes. Some amniotic fluid had dropped on his foot. The porter caught up with him.

"Ba Sir, I have truly respected you. You are a great man. You did a caesarean in just seven minutes. Actually, it was six by my watch; this is unbelievable. I see Caesars lasting two hours in this theatre. I always wondered what they cut inside these poor women's interiors," Mr. Yikolo told Marx. "Some Caesareans, I have witnessed in this theatre, last ninety minutes like a football match."

"Really, that's bad," Marx answered. "Promise me you won't go out and tell people what you witnessed here tonight.

Meanwhile in theatre, the team discussed what they just witnessed among themselves.

"The student didn't even see anything," the anesthetist remarked.

"Did you see the movement in his hands? It was like magic," the midwife remarked.

"You saw that; I thought you were sleeping. What was the delivery time?" the anesthetist laughed at the midwife.

"Get lost; the baby was born within seconds. I just blinked and next I saw was the baby," the midwife answered.

"I have worked with many surgeons in my thirty five years of theatre nursing. But I have never seen anyone with fluid hands like this. He was like someone stroking the wind. I am still amazed by what has just happened here," she explained to her equally mesmerized team.

The baby was crying and looked out of immediate danger from asphyxia. However, it had a high risk for developing sepsis. Marx returned to the operating room to face a barrage of questions.

"Doctor, who are you? Where are you from? What do you do? We have never seen anything like this," the midwife asked in total amusement.

"We will be sending for you every night when we have a case. You will save us from long standing hours," the coverage nurse remarked.

Marx smiled "I was invited to share these skills with your doctors. Unfortunately everyone has taken a holiday now that I am here."

"How could they do that? These skills would have benefited the community here and the hospital. A Caesarean section under ten minutes, who wouldn't want to learn that?" the midwife asked still dazed by '*Maximusement*'.

"That is ACH doctors for you," said the anaesthetist.

"My best time yet was five minutes," said Marx.

"Start to finish," Joan sort clarification.

"Yes my dear, start to finish. However, I have vowed never to routinely push a caesarean to less than seven minutes," he said.

"Why not below seven minutes, when it is possible?" Jessica asked.

"Because then it becomes a sport. And when many begin to try to break my record or attempt to set their own records, patients will die. These are dangerous skills to place in people's hands. With great skills comes greater responsibility," Marx cautioned his students.

He left the hospital past midnight after passing through the wards to check on Rhoda and Moses. Deep inside his heart, he was enjoying the beautiful company Jessica and Joan presented him. He found himself fighting the desires of his flesh. He thought Joan had looked at him with longing eyes on the operating table. He resisted burning enticement to elope with her to his cold room at the Inn.

Thoughts and visions he had no control over where rolling inside his mind. He saw her wrapped around his cold body at the Inn. She was smiling and tickling him. He wondered what thoughts ran in the minds of the girls running around the wards with him at midnight. He was sure they would flee if they saw his weird thoughts at that hour. The girls' beauty had turned Marx's exhausted brain delusional. He knew at that moment, he needed to flee the hospital. He blamed his earthly desires on his exhausted lonely brain. It had been a long day.

***

Anything but Duty before Self

The sun was shining outside beckoning him to rise and join in. This was his first Saturday in Mbala. He lay in bed reflecting over his work. "What an incredible week it has been," he murmured to himself.

He wanted to get up but Newton's first law of motion prevented him from escaping his rugged bed at the Inn. He recited the law to himself, "an object at rest stays at rest and an object in motion stays in motion with the same speed and in the same direction unless acted upon by an unbalanced force." He remained pinned to his bed like an object Newton had referred to.

"I am not an object," he spoke to himself. "Objects have no brains, they cannot think. Sorry Newton, I cannot obey your law. Your law should state, an object without a brain stays at rest or in motion…"

Just then, there was a knock at the door. He wondered who it could be as he sprung to his feet to open the door. His heart sunk when he found it was the lady at the reception. He had hoped to see Joan's beautiful face standing at the door.

"Sorry to disturb you sir, I came to tell you that the restaurant is closed today," she said.

"What do you mean closed?" he asked.

"It is Saturday today sir, the owner of this Inn is SDA," she tried to explain.

"What is SDA? What has it got to do with my food?" he asked rubbing his sleepy eyes.

"Seventh Day Adventist Church sir," she answered smiling. "They don't cook on Saturday. It is a sin."

"What? Don't you think that is silly?" he remarked. "I think it is a greater sin to starve your guests."

"I am merely an employee sir," she answered.

This gave Marx an idea; he would visit an SDA church that morning to find out what these folks who were starving him did.

After a hot shower, he strode to the road side to take a taxi. A pleasant young fellow called Shing'onga picked him.

"Muli uli ba sir *(how are you sir)*?" he greeted Marx as was the custom by Taxi drivers here. Marx found them extremely courteous.

"Nili Ningo, thank you. Take me to an SDA church," he answered.

"Which one in particular sir?" he asked.

"I don't know any. Take me to any; where common people go," he said.

"There are four SDA churches here. I will take you to central church. It is their best and was recently built. The floors are tiled and church is spacious. You will love it there," Shing'onga explained excitedly.

"No, not there," Marx declined Shing'onga's suggested place of worship. "Places like those are likely to be patronized by self opinionated individuals. I don't want where pompous people love to go. I want where I can find genuine and down to earth people of Mbala."

"In that case, I know just the right place for you Ba Sir," Shing'onga beamed with excitement. "I will take you to old Location, near the old market. There is an old SDA church there."

He stepped on the gas pedal after making a left turn at the First World War memorial round about. This was the place where General Von Lettow- Vorbeck formally surrendered on 25th November, 1918. This memorial site was designed by Sir Edwin Lutyens.

"I am taking you to Lucheche SDA church Ba Sir, you will find wonderful and humble people there sir." Shing'onga announced steering his corolla along a bumpy dirt road.

Soon, they came to a bridge where some road works had been done to elevate the bridge. On the right, a Chinese construction company had set camp. Heavy machinery and construction vehicles could be seen over a small fence. Marx found the site very strategic and foolish. It was close to a river they had just crossed. This stream would provide the construction workers unlimited source of proteins. The river had an abundant frog and snake species waiting to make the menu on the contractor's dining table.

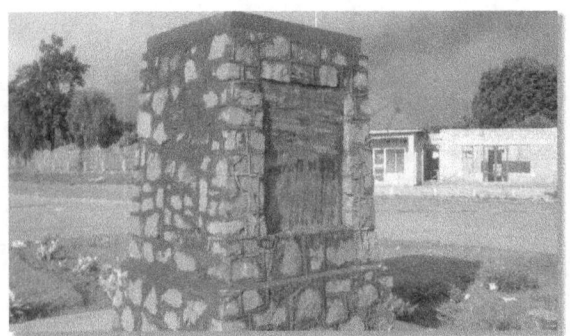

This was also a malaria breeding ground. With the high prevalence of malaria in Mbala, Marx was certain this river would feed and slay numerous construction workers by the time the roads were done. He recommended setting up a malaria and trauma clinic on site.

While, he was thinking these things, they drove through an old market. Several vendors stood by their stands hoping the Taxi would come to a stop on their door. They would never know, the passenger on this Taxi, was in their area for quite a different business agenda.

***

Lucheche SDA church was a humble place of worship. However, it was not the kind of humbleness Marx had hoped for. The people dressed immaculate and spoke good English. The usher received Marx at the door and led him to a VIP section of the church. He stopped when his quick mind scanned the area he was being guiding to. He broke away from his guide and sat himself to a crowded humble section. The church was full. A choir sung at the altar. Marx could not remember the last time he was in church.

He sat in awe admiring the décor at the altar. It was decorated in beautiful and colorful fluorescent blue and yellow frilled curtains. The designer the church had hired truly knew his trade. He forgave them for denying him food at the Inn. While he was 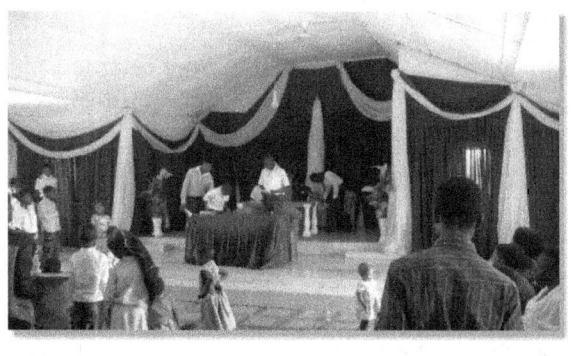 still absorbing the interior and running spot diagnoses on the congregants, Marx's phone rang. It was the hospital calling. He rushed outside to take the call. One of the elders followed Marx outside.

"Is everything alright sir," he asked when Marx had put down his phone.

Marx was startled. He hadn't noticed someone was standing behind him.

"There is an emergency at the hospital. They are sending transport in twenty minutes," he answered.

"An Emergency; let me take you there. Come, my car is over there," the Church elder suggested walking to his car. "My name is Ephraim; I am the owner of Giza Inn."

"Really, I am staying at Giza Inn. What a pleasant surprise," Marx remarked. He wanted to complain about the restaurant; however he chose to keep quiet on the matter.

"I am certain God planned for us to meet like this. The favour of God is upon you," the church elder explained.

They left Lucheche SDA church and drove to Abercorn Community Hospital. Marx was touched by the action taken by this church elder. His mind shifted to ponder on the case waiting for him at ACH. The nurse had sounded anxious. The patient had been referred from the Air Force clinic with a retained placenta. The experienced midwives at ACH attempted to deliver the placenta but failed. The patient was bleeding profusely when they called. Marx gave her a working diagnosis of PPH. This was by far the leading cause of maternal death in Zambia.

"I have no doubt doc; this is a retained placenta and atonic uterus. She may even have a ruptured uterus. Unfortunately, we have no blood in the hospital or other plasma expanders. Her BP is un-recordable doc," the nurse had explained anxiously over the phone.

PPH is abbreviation for Postpartum Hemorrhage. It is a term used to refer to excessive bleeding after delivery. This condition is responsible for the death of numerous women in Zambia, particularly in rural areas where Marx was. The risk factors for PPH include; Retained placenta or incomplete evacuation of placenta after delivery, injury in the birth canal during delivery, injury of the womb including tears or rapture of the Uterus, Atonic Uterus;

Uterine Atony is seen in women who have had many children or high parity, over-distension of the womb during pregnancy such as in multi foetal pregnancies, Diabetes in pregnancy; some anesthetic drugs, clotting disorders etc…

Atonic Uterus refers to failure by the womb to contract or harden after delivery. When this happens it can lead to massive bleeding referred to as PPH; and place the life of a woman in jeopardy. Hemorrhage remains the leading cause of death among mothers in Zambia.

A hardened womb soon after delivery causes significant lower abdominal discomfort and back ache. Many women complain about this when they ought to rejoice. This is a sign of Life. A woman who does not feel this pain should get worried as this may be an early warning of impending doom; the exception being women given adequate analgesics soon after delivery. When excess bleeding occurs, a woman starts to feel dizzy, her heart starts to beat very fast and she may feel air around her to be insufficient. If she is made to stand and/or walk, she may lose consciousness and fall down. And if there is no urgent medical help, a woman may die.

When they arrived at the hospital, Marx hurriedly bade farewell to the Church elder and splinted to the Labour ward. He found the mid wives exhausted. The patient lay in a pool of blood on the bed dying.

Dr Marximillian introduced himself to the patient and once he had her consent, he hurriedly got a pair of gynecological gloves and hastily guided his large hand into the patient's birth canal. He reached the cervix and pushed his hand further upwards to enter the uterus.

The mid wives sat on stools watching. They were sure Dr Marximillian would fail too. They had snapped the umbilical cord in their earlier attempt to deliver this killer placenta. However the evil placenta refused to let go.

Marx felt his way inside the uterus and soon found a stable point to haul on. He gently worked his hand using every trick he had learnt as an OBG resident. His left hand gently steadied the Uterus via the abdomen. Shortly, he gently withdraw his hand from the birth canal with the placenta following. Seeing this, the midwife spontaneously sprung to their feet and gave Dr Marximillian a standing ovation.

Several nurses had gathered to watch Dr Marximillian at work; as where several Medical students; Felix, Kaoma, Kaluba, Joy, Johnny, Jessy, Joan, Jessica, O'Neil and Ethel.

"This is unbelievable, how did you do it?" a midwife asked.

"We have never failed to remove a placenta before in this labour ward. This was a strange placenta," the coverage nurse remarked.

"We have never met a stubborn placenta such as this one. How did you do it?" a senior mid wife asked.

"It wasn't me," Marx answered vaguely with a grin on his face.

"But we all saw you Doctor," a nurse commented with a puzzled look on her face.

"God sent his angels to remove it. When you called me, I was in church. I was certain we would end up operating going by the description you gave me over the phone," Dr Marximillian explained.

Marx left everyone in labour ward wondering who he truly was. He was quickly becoming legend at ACH. Some said he was a Surgeon. Others insisted he was an Obstetrician. While others said he was a man sent to their hospital by God. They didn't know Marx was a mere mortal made of flesh and blood. He was in deep debt like so many of them. A mere man rubbished by the System to be a fake and a scoundrel, whom they were hounding and haranguing with smiles on their spiteful faces;

**

He left for the Gyn ward to check on his patient Rhoda. It was nearly 1 pm by now. His patient didn't look too well. She was severely anemic. Her hemoglobin had dropped to 4g/dl. Her legs were swollen and she looked puffy on the face. The cut down wounds on her ankle joints were getting infected. The day of the operation, Marx had been called to the hospital at night to perform a cut down as the doctor on call could not establish a venous access in the usual way.

There was still no blood at ACH. She was dying from anemia and organ failure. The nearest hospital where a pint of blood could be found was one thousand kilometers away.

Seeing her condition had deteriorated further, the relatives approached Marx and requested to take their patient home. However, the nurses advised Marx not to let them go. They warned him, she would end up at a traditional doctor's kraal. Her best chance of survival was in the hospital where there was still a glitter of hope blood would be sent from the central point in the capital. After counseling Rhoda's relatives, Marx left the hospital.

***

He strode towards town to search for a restaurant. He was very hungry. Several eating places where closed owing to it being a Sabbath. After a long walk, he came to a large building named Ten Kwacha. Dark rain clouds were gathering in the sky above.

He stood for a while wondering why it was so named. However, he was too hungry to launch an inquiry at that moment. Several call boys stood in the wide corridors of Ten Kwacha. Marx stepped inside and ordered a meal which he hurriedly ate in the corner of a spacious dinning. He thought the light was too dim for him to see clearly. He couldn't even see his meal clearly. "Maybe the chef wants to conceal something in the soup," he thought to himself. It was 4 pm when he left Ten Kwacha restaurant.

He stood in the corridor for a while. Several women were selling dry Sardines and others were roasting Cassava.

A large bus was loading passengers just across to where he stood. He recognized the bus immediately; this was the bus he had ridden on from Lusaka. And it was at this bus station he had resisted the temptation to ask Ms Isaacs to accompany him to his 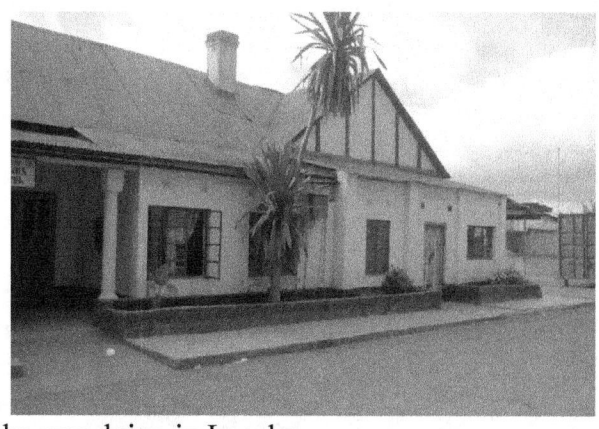 Lodge. He wondered how she was doing in Lusaka.

While he thought these things, a huge deluge came upon the town. It rained cats and dogs over ten kwacha. Pools of water collected all around bringing to light the poor drainage in the area.

Marx left Ten Kwacha to seek shelter at the magnificent Victorian building next door. This was the famous Arms Hotel. Marx admired its Architectural design. He was received by a beautiful receptionist. She showed him the interior and rooms of the hotel. However, she proved to be very ignorant about the history of the magnificent hotel and failed to lure Marx into trading his cold room at Giza for a cozy room at the Arms hotel. He was deeply disappointed with her. He loved the look of the spacious Bar. The buffalo head on the wall stared angrily at him. 'It must have presided over many drunken confrontations among the bar's patrons in the fifties and sixties,' he thought.

The Beatles must have played here. The Large Chimney protruding on the roof still looked as elegant as it did more than a century earlier.

Several travelers stood in the hotel lobby. They were waiting for buses that used the hotel premises as a bus station. Marx's heart sunk when he learnt, his bravura hotel had been turned into an intercity bus station.

He recalled seeing a picture taken in 1958, of three magnificent MGs that had parked there in route to Cape Town from Cairo. This little picture gave Marx a glimpse into the importance Mbala must have played to Trans Africa Travelers in those days. They stopped and refreshed at the Arms hotel and watered their perched throats with the finest beer sold in the Hotel Bar. The place where the MGs had poised was now a parking lot for taxis and large buses en route to distant towns in Zambia.

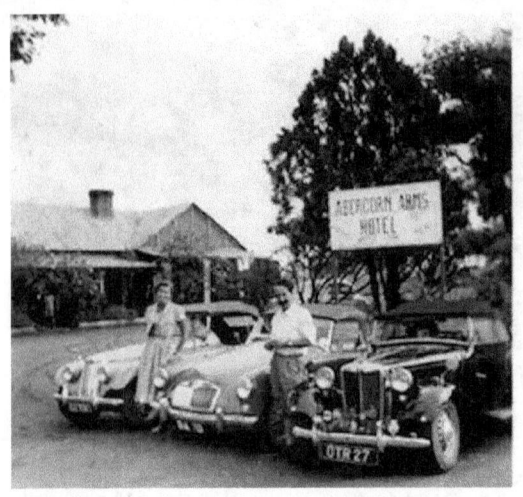

Soon the rain let off as suddenly as it had begun. He considered calling Ms Isaacs on his phone as he strode down President Avenue towards the First World War Memorial. Marx walked down the road humming a survival song, clicking his fingers and nodding his head back and forth. He knew he could not depend on others for his happiness. He searched his own heart to light a candle of joy. (The magnificent MGs poise at the Arms Hotel in 1958)

I'm a survivor
I'm not gonna give up
I'm not gon' stop
I'm gonna move on
And survive
I'm gonna make it
I will survive
I'm not gonna give up
I'm not gon' stop

Now that you have exterminated my pay
I'm so much better
You thought I'd be vulnerable without it
But I'm stronger
You thought I'd be a drifter without a salary
But I'm richer
You thought that I'd be sad without pay
I laugh harder
You thought that debt would stress me
It gave me a new birth
You conspired to take away my earnings
But I'm chilling
You thought that I'd fail to Care
I'm more compassionate now
I'm as loving to the sick as I have always been
I'm wiser
I'm smarter now

And I know this shit is all about the money

I'm a survivor
I'm not gonna give up
I'm not gon' stop
I'm gonna move on
And survive
I'm gonna make it
I will survive
I'm not gonna give up
I'm not gon' stop

Just so you know
I have had too much fun to call what I do work
When God closes a door
He opens a window

Clouds raced in the sky above. The weather was chilly and somewhat windy. There were few people on the road. A lady in a blue dress hurried down the road three meters ahead of Marx. In front of her, a girl in a stylish skirt, he estimated to be around eleven hurried in the same direction balancing a heavy yellow bucket full of sugarcane on her head.

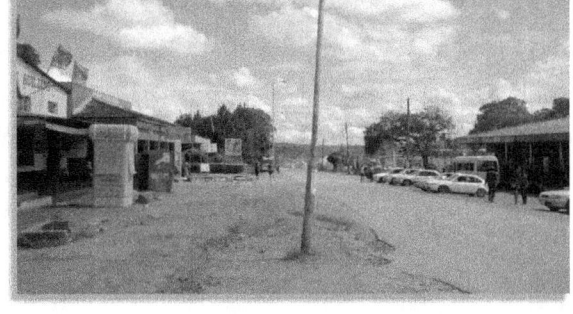

He passed a Gas service station on his right and walked leisurely down the brown tarred road. An office building belonging to the Zambia electricity company in the area on his right looked deserted. He couldn't see anyone inside working. However, he thought they had done a wonderful job in Mbala as there were no power cuts ever since he arrived.

Dr Marximillian had forgotten it was a weekend. His thought process was interrupted momentarily when a woman in a blue Jean trouser greeted him. She was headed in the opposite direction and carried a baby on her back. He thought she had probably seen him at the hospital.

He then turned his mind to reflect on how babies survive. 'They are born attached to an umbilicus,' he thought.

At birth, the baby is separated from its umbilicus in the most pitiless manner imaginable. Marx considered the whole birthing practice to be a brutal process and one that had power to kill. He found he could draw parallels to his present predicaments.

At birth, a baby comes equipped with an armory of alternative umbilici. The mouth is the most noticeable food portal to use when the baby leaves the aquarium of the womb.

Humans were never created to be mono-umbilicus creatures. Food is a primary survival resource. All else; eyes, legs, hands, ears etc help man find and defend his food. Humans switch to a convenient and most appropriate umbilicus depending on the environment they find themselves in. Hostile environments such as the aquariums in a mother's wombs

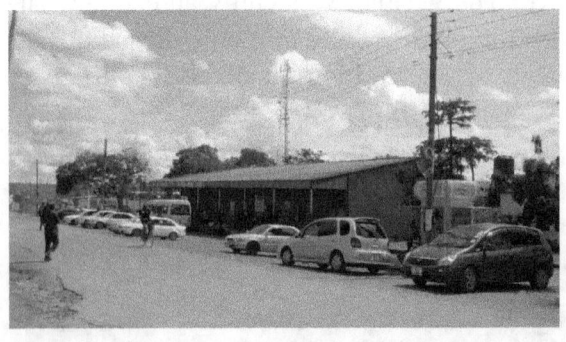

require a longer and flexible cord attached to their abdomens like astronauts.

At birth, humans face an even more hostile environment requiring them to have several umbilici or portals. One port is dedicated to liquids and solids; the other portal is for capturing air; and another for sound. A separate portal is needed to capture light, the hallmark of vision.

Then there are those portals man brags less about; they handle waste disposal. Complex earthly machines, such as man, got to produce waste. It is a paradox that the portals for pleasure should be intricately fused with those for waste disposal. These orifices or portals make humans multi-umbilici. This is all for the purpose of survival.

Babies are born engineered for survival, so is everyone. However, man is not born once, each time he faces turmoil and shake up in his life, a rebirth takes place. He is ushered into a new world by a re-birth unlike a biological one; when he survives it, that is.

A street vendor in Cairo road once told Marx, 'when you read a book, you become a different person. The book changes you. You are not the same person you where in chapter one.'

Marx realized he had kept all his eggs in one basket far too long; he had over trusted *The System*. He had placed his earthly duty before self. At the height of the Zimbabwean Economic Meltdown, the citizens had coined a popular survival slogan; 'It is better to lose Zimbabwe than to lose the World.' Dr Marximillian found this expression extremely intriguing. It was better to lose his dedication to work than to lose himself.

* * *

Several forces of evil had conspired against Marx. He was thrown in the abyss of debt by wicked people. The only crime he had committed was to be innovative and take a risk at a start up business. His country was in debt from senseless borrowing; however it was not being harangued by its lenders as he was. When banks crushed during the global financial meltdown, they pleaded for bailout to save them from failing.

The System and lenders chose to impose a financial embargo on Marx instead of a bailout plan. The court initiated a scandalous scheme against him. Marx wondered what interest the court had in punishing him like a criminal. He was sure his evil midget judge had austere motives in minting out this harsh judgment. He took 95% from Marx's meager pay and gave it to his Chez Ntemba escort. Marx was left to survive on 5%. All maids in the hospital were now earning a salary higher than Dr Marximillian. He could not afford to buy food, let alone support his mother, orphans in his care and send money to his lovely children. He could no longer pay rentals on time making his land lords extremely impatient. A learned doctor had just been thrown on the streets by a stupid and misguided court order.

* * *

A week earlier, misdirectors at *The System's* position filing resource sat in their offices and decided Marx's fate via online chat.

Officers entrusted with making the work place a pleasurable experience were delighted to inflict financial doom on Dr Marximillian. They conspired in their offices on how they would enforce the outrageous court order. No one was thinking about offering solutions that would bail out Marx and keep him at work. As far as they were concerned, this was simply a case to be filed and a position to be filled when it fell vacant. They wrote each other flowery confidential texts. Luckily, Marx was kept informed by a few good men and women in the establishment.

"I have an interesting court order for you to see," one Misdirector wrote on an encrypted chat platform.

"What case is it about?" Misdirected asked.

"File MH370; It is about these fellows paid too much money while we do the donkey work," Misdirector answered.

"A fellow called Marximillian; file MH370," Misdirected recalled the issue.

"Yes, I will send you the court order. Please enforce it with pleasure. I don't care whether he quits," said Misdirector.

"For you, I will make him regret ever joining this ministry. We have many foreign doctors who can take his job and do it even better," Misdirected obliged.

"You know," Misdirector remarked.

"I will ensure accounts takes out 99% from his earnings," Misdirected promised. "I'll make him pay for his sins. I'll enforce IMF like austerity measures. He will fire himself by the time I am through with him."

"Keep this confidential; it is from an unscrupulous court Judge. I think he is benefiting from this," Misdirector advised his collaborator.

"With pleasure," Misdirected agreed.

"I hate these Local doctors. I find them impertinent, brazen, impudent, blatant, insolent, cheeky, impolite, arrogant and presumptuous. If I had my way, I would send all of them to the streets and replace them with Congolese and Chinese doctors. We pay them too much money. On their salary, we can employ five Chinese doctors," Misdirector remarked.

"We employ three thousand doctors. This would translate to fifteen thousand dedicated Chinese doctors or even thirty thousand, without any increased expense from the treasury. Incredible what simple ratios and smart computing can achieve," Misdirected agreed.

"Local doctors are too expensive. They are uneconomical for the country. They take up large spaces in our limited position filing resources. We ought to share this scarce cake equally. We shouldn't allow one cadre stream fill up all our limited positions," they chattered endlessly.

***

While Marx worked day and night at ACH, forces of evil lurked all around and conspired against him. They came out of demon holes in their millions. He was unaware about this online conspiracy. He had just spent his last penny at Ten Kwacha restaurant and had no idea his salary would never come.

The weather was pleasant outside. It was slightly windy though. Marx understood why the British Colonial Administrators favoured this area, calling it Healthy and describing it as having a pleasant climate. Besides being suitable for living, Abercorn as it was known presented the British settlers an abundance of Hunting and Fishing activities. When the British South Africa Company took over administration of the territory in 1895, operating as the African Lakes Company, they called it North-Eastern Rhodesia and the 'Zombe Boma' became known as Abercorn, named after the company chairman.

The sun hovered low on the western horizon, giving it an orange red glow. Dusk was taking over the small town of Mbala. He walked leisurely along President Avenue. Several cars lined up to refuel at a yellow service station down the road. Many were preparing to drive off to distant destinations.

He was exhausted when he got to his room at the Inn. It was now 6pm.

His mind was weary. He was sure; he had become a danger to his patients. He needed to go on a long vacation from his work.

He decided to pray, hoping this would ease his mind. He knelt by his bed;

"My Father in heaven," he said.
"Hallowed be your name.
Please do not let me fall in the hands my enemies.
Forgive my sins
Do not treat me as my sins deserve.

Forgive me I pray
Vengeance is yours O' Lord
If my suffering is an act of man
I pray may the wrath of God fall on them be it so severely
Forgive me for asking the destruction of my enemies
Vengeance is yours
I forgive all my enemies
Forgive me my debts as I have forgiven my debtors
Deliver me from the evil one
If my suffering is an act of Satan
Please deliver me from Satan and his demons
If my suffering is of my own making
I lay it on your feet
Give me a lighter York to carry
Deliver me
Please open my eyes,
Grant me wisdom to come out of this trap
If my suffering is by the hand of God
Please forgive my sins
I am merely a man of flesh and blood
There is no place I can ran to
There is no where I can hide from your wrath
Save me like many patients you have healed under my care
I have seen you save many people whom you sent me to
I witnessed your healing hand many times
You are a healing God
Please do not hide your face from me
Forgive my sins
Heal me O' Lord
Deliver me from my Enemies

I know a physician is not angry at the intemperance of a mad patient, nor does he take it ill to be railed at by a man in fever. Just so should a wise man treat all mankind, as a physician does his patient, and look upon them only as sick and extravagant.

I thank you because you hear my prayer

Marx fell asleep on his knees at the edge of his bed. He was worn out.

It had become very clear to him, he couldn't continue working. He needed to take another path in his life. He knew however, it would be very hard for him to leave behind the only thing he knew best, caring for his patients. Nonetheless, he was willing to try out new things and learn to care for himself. Over the years, he had neglected his own life. He thought very little about his own welfare. It was time now, he took care of himself. He knew he wasn't indispensable. "After all, there would always be the sick in the world," he reminded himself.

Later that night at 11pm, he was awoken by a loud knock at his door. He sprung to his feet wondering who it could be at such a late hour. His phone was switched off. When he got to the door, he found the driver anxiously standing outside.

"Sorry to disturb you boss. You are wanted at the hospital," he said.

Dr Marximillian stood staring at the driver for a while. He was struggling not to vent his frustration on the poor fellow standing at the door. A gentle breeze blew into his face and calmed his tempestuous mind.

"The coverage nurse said she tried your number but wasn't going through," the driver tried to explain.

"Give me a minute," Marx closed his door leaving the poor fellow outside confused.

***

The patient they were calling Dr Marximillian for had come from Kawimbe, a village on the border between Zambia and Tanzania. She had fallen off a motor bike on the way to hospital. She had booked a motor cyclist to take her to hospital with her mother. Unfortunately on the way, they had an accident and she fell off. The motor cyclist had carried too many people on his motor bike. Three grown women were more than he could manage. To make matters worse, the alcohol he had consumed gravely impaired his ability to negotiate the treacherous path to ACH. She arrived at the hospital bleeding from the womb. The midwives gave her a working diagnosis of APH. She reported to the nurses that they had fallen off the motor bike three times when the 'driver' lost control. She told the nurses he had been drinking when he picked them. The nurses feared she could have abruption placenta. They asked the coverage nurse to send for Dr Marximillian immediately. The baby was severely distressed and needed urgent caesarean section.

Dr Marximillian arrived in theatre and found his patient already on the operating table.

"I hope you didn't have to wait very long," he asked reading the faces of the team in theatre.

"No, the patient has just arrived," the anesthetist answered.

"How is the foetal heart? He asked.

"Still present; the last one I took was 180," the midwife answered.

Dr Marximillian got the foetal scope and listened for the heart beat himself. He didn't like what he heard. The baby was in serious trouble. It needed a miracle to survive.

***

As soon as the theatre nurse was ready, Marx scrubbed in and was soon standing on the operating table. The mid wife was ready with the baby towel. Word about Dr Marximillian's Guinness caesarean records had reached her. She wasn't taking any chances and be caught fumbling when the baby was delivered.

"I want to see how you do your caesareans. Last time I didn't see a thing," the theatre nurse remarked.

"Just ensure you don't blink," Dr Marximillian answered smiling.

So saying, he picked the knife and with a magical stroke, he opened the patient's abdomen in the usual way.

Before the theatre nurse, could let out the words, 'starting time', Marx had opened the uterus and delivered a cute female baby. He passed her to the midwife who was still spell bound by what she had witnessed. The caesarean section was over within seven minutes and Marx stepped out of the operating table.

"Dr Marximillian, this is impossible," the theatre nurse remarked deeply amazed.

"I agree dear," he answered.

"How on earth do you do it?" the midwife asked wrapping the baby in a warm blanket.

"It wasn't me alone; we did this together. This team did this extraordinary operation and saved this baby," he answered.

"How did you do it? I saw your hands, they were incredible. I can't describe what I was seeing," the coverage nurse remarked.

"It was dictated by the emergency of this situation. This baby needed this timely intervention to survive. I am afraid this maybe my last operation," he said.

"What? Are you leaving us already?" the anesthetist asked.

"I am still here. There are, however, people who think I shouldn't continue working," he said vaguely.

He left the operating room for the male change room. The team remained puzzled by his comment. They couldn't figure out which people Marx was referring to. It was now twenty minutes past midnight. He was hungry. His Ten Kwacha meal had a very short half live. However, he was not in a hurry to get back to his room at the Inn.

He decided to take a stroll to the surgical wards and check on his patient Moses. He ran into a beautiful young nurse. She was the chief's daughter.

"What are you doing here?" he asked her

"I am volunteering my time," she answered.

"The chief's daughter doesn't need to work," he replied. "She ought to be learning how to run the kingdom."

"She also needs to learn to stand on her own two feet. She must learn not to depend on others for her happiness," she replied looking Marx in the eye.

"Wow, impressive. She has a brain," he smiled candidly at her.

"I have a degree in social work and a diploma in Nursing," she smiled back at him.

She led him into the nurse's station where they sat down. Marx gave her the feeling as though they had met before.

"Why do I feel like we have met before?" she asked him when they sat down.

"It is called Déjà Vu. I was about to ask the same question," he answered looking at her.

"How did you know I was the chief's daughter then?" she asked surprised.

"I didn't know," he replied.

"You asked what the chief's daughter was doing when you walked into this ward a while ago," she insisted.

"You are a princess, I am pleased to make your acquaintance," he answered.

"Stop playing with my mind. I think you truly know who I am," she said firmly.

"Princess Fiona, this is no game and I don't mean to offend you. I am here to check on my patient. Let me see him and I will be on my way. I wouldn't want to disturb the harmony of your kingdom," he answered getting up to leave.

"I am sorry; Don't leave, I didn't mean to get angry. I have a few things troubling my mind. Can you forgive me?" she said sitting on a sofa next to him. "You can call me Isabelle."

"Pleased to meet you Isabelle, I am Dr Marximillian. You can call me Marx; I want to visit Mpulungu harbor tomorrow, I would be pleased if you came with me," said Marx.

"You mean today or Monday tomorrow. I would love to; I could use an escape to the harbor, however you would need to disguise me if I came with you. Everyone knows my parents in this town," she answered.

Retreat Royale

Eight hours later at 10am, Marx eloped with the Chief's daughter. They drove to Mpulungu chatting the entire way. They were like two people that had met before. She was 23 and incredibly beautiful. She wore a beautiful perfume that tickled Marx's olfactory apparatus the entire trip.

"You told me you came by bus from Lusaka. Whose car is this?" she asked as they drove passed an Air force base.

"Do you like it? It belongs to an old friend of mine. He is out to Lusaka," he answered.

She thought for a while and stared through the window in deep thought. Marx noticed.

"I love the weather in Mbala. It feels like Europe here. Look at the grass, it is still green. In my town, you can even torch it this time of the year," he said stealing a glance at her. He didn't want to probe into her personal space. It was too early to let skeletons out of the cupboard.

"Mpulungu is not like Mbala. It will be hot there," she said looking thoughtfully at Marx. "Why do I feel so free and comfortable with you?"

"I don't know. Maybe I remind you of someone. Fellows with multiple personalities resemble everyone. Try to remember who it is. I hope it isn't an ex boyfriend, because I will hunt him down and punish him for hurting you," he answered smiling warmly at her.

"Actually yes," she answered laughing. "How did you know? You seem to know quite a lot about me. I am suspicious."

"No way, say you are joking," said Marx looking straight at her. "Where is he?"

"He doesn't want to see me anymore. My parents rejected the plates he sent to ask for my hand," She said looking outside the window. "They told me to find someone intelligent with a respectable job."

"I am sorry to hear that," said Marx and resisted to ask probing questions. He was aware how vulnerable a broken heart could be.

"Look, that is Lunzuwa power station over there," she pointed to the mountains on their left.

Marx slowed the explorer they were travelling in and brought it to a halt on the road side to catch a glimpse of the power station. He couldn't see any buildings.

"Where is it?" he asked stepping out of the car.

"Over there where there is a water fall," she said when he had opened the door for her. "It used to produce only 0.75 megawatts, but now produces 14.8 megawatts after a $52 million upgrade.

"That explains why there are no power cuts in Mbala," said Marx reflecting on the worst power cuts the rest of the country was facing. "In my town, we have power cuts daily lasting up to 12 hours at a time. I think I will shift to Mbala."

"You should shift right now," she smiled warmly at him.

They stood like lovers and leaned against the side of the Ford Explorer. Marx considered turning to face her and kiss the chief's daughter and pin her against their vehicle. He had watched too many movies and some scenes he had seen where now conspiring against him to do the same. "I don't want to be charged with indecent assault and sexual harassment. She is too vulnerable," he mumbled to himself.

"What are you saying?" she asked.

"I was saying this scenery looks very beautiful. Look at the blue mountains in the distance," he lied.

"I love it. My father has a farm somewhere beyond those Blue Mountains. Strange, I feel happy standing with a stranger in the mountains," she said.

"A stranger you met at mid night on the ward, ten hours ago," he smiled opening the passenger door for her. Their eyes met. She quickly looked down. His heart started to beat fast.

"I don't want to go. Leave me here," she said smiling.

"I won't let wild animals eat you. I will erect two tents and light a fire in that case. You can fetch some firewood and water while I hunt deer for our dinner," he remarked.

"Deer will take you a long way into the forest. Wild animals will eat you. Just gather some roots, leaves and tubers. Include some Fruits and Mushrooms," she smiled walking towards the door.

"Mm hunter gatherer; I am afraid, I lost all those skills. The only skills I have left are for the supermarket, where I can easily pick leaves, tubers, mushrooms and chocolates with easy. Out here, the supermarket of the jungle is treacherous. We will be picked cold and lifeless from mushroom poisoning," he laughed as they drove off.

"Why couldn't he be like you?" she asked.

"Each person is amazing, funny and mysterious in their own unique way," he said as they drove up a mountain road.

"Look over there; that is Lake Tanganyika. I love this view very much," she said pointing at the blue scenery in the distance.

They had arrived in Mpulungu and the weather changed instantly. It was hot; the temperature was 43 degrees centigrade. They left Mbala at 14.2 degrees. The roads where neatly paved in town unlike those in Mbala.

"Who is the area member of parliament here? He has done an incredible job. The roads look pretty. I am sure the people will vote for him again. I would vote for him too," Marx remarked admiring the town roads.

"I heard he is not standing. Something to do with some certificates recently enshrined in the constitution," she said.

"I think these roads are a better certificate. This is equivalent to a degree in town planning and civil engineering," said Marx as they passed a busy trading post. "Which way is the harbor?"

"Drive straight ahead. I think it is closed today, but I can talk to someone to let us in," she said excitedly.

They drove down a slope and soon stopped in front of an old black gate. They had arrived at the harbor.

***

They were received inside by a cheerful man in his late forties. He led them to the water edge where a large vessel was docked in port.

"Welcome to Mpulungu Port," he said. "The princess has informed me you are a doctor. I am pleased to meet you."

"On Sundays, like today, I am a tourist," said Marx wondering when the chief's daughter made the introductions. She smiled when their eyes met. She was walking towards the large cargo ship in port.

"Have you ever been to Mpulungu before?" Mr. Simfukwe, the port official asked.

"This is my first time. I have always wanted to visit this place," he answered. "I have always wondered where the name Mpulungu was derived from."

Mr. Simfukwe turned to their left and pointed at a large mountain near to where they stood, "This is Mpulungu. Behind this mountain, the Lungu people traded with Arab slave traffickers. They would say to the Arabs, *'Mpa Ulungu, nkumpe chi mwana chi Bwalya na chi nshupa. Senda Bwalya, Ine mpa Ulungu,'* literary meaning, give me beads, I give you this child, Bwalya, he is a trouble maker."

"So *Mpa Ulungu* became *Mpulungu,*" Marx's quick mind made the connection.

"Exactly, that's how we ended up with this name. During the colonial era though, this place was called Tanganyika. But because of a similar name in Tanzania, it was changed to Mpulungu when Zambia attained independence from British rule. The name Tanganyika is derived from *Tanganika* which refers to; *the great lake spreading out like a plain."* he explained. "Lake Tanganyika is Africa's Greatest Lake. It is the longest fresh water lake in the world."

Marx recalled what he knew about this great lake from his geography class in junior high. Most of it had faded away from his memory. It had been many years since, however he still remembered this was the second largest fresh water lake in the world by volume and that it was the second deepest, in both cases, after only Lake Baikal in Siberia, Russia.

"Four countries share Lake Tanganyika; Zambia, Tanzania, Burundi and Congo DRC," Mr. Simfukwe lectured on with karate like gestures, pointing repeatedly at the great lake in front of them. "This Lake is situated within the Albertine Rift, the western branch of the East African Rift and is confined by the mountainous walls of the valley. It is the largest rift lake in Africa and is the deepest lake in Africa. It holds the greatest volume of fresh water, accounting for 18% of the world's available fresh water. It stretches for 676 km in a general north - south direction. It has a catchment area of 231,000 square kilometers. Due to the Lake's Tropical location, it suffers a high rate of evaporation. Thus, it depends on a high inflow through the Ruziz out of Lake Kivu to keep the lake high enough to overflow. It has one major outflow, the Lukanga River which empties into the Congo River drainage. The Malagarasi River, which is Tanzania's second largest river, enters the lake on the eastern side. This river is older than Lake Tanganyika. Before the Lake was formed, the Malagarasi used to drain directly into River Congo."

"676 km, that's the distance from Mpulungu to Serenje," Marx remarked amused by the incredible length of the Lake he was looking at, "I wonder how the lake would have influenced our way of life in Zambia if we didn't have to share it with anyone. I am sure I would have traveled by ship from Serenje to Mbala."

"We wouldn't feel like a land locked country. We would all have become great Marinas," Mr. Simfukwe agreed with Marx. "I am sure had the lake been entirely Zambian waters, Fishing would have been the major economic activity in Northern and part of Central Zambia."

Lake Tanganyika played an important role during the First World War. In the early years of the war, the Germans had total control of the lake. In recent history, the celebrated Argentinean revolutionary, Che Guevara used the western shores of the Lake as a training camp for guerrilla forces in the Congo.

"Global warming has taken a toll on the lake," Mr. Simfukwe explained with obvious worry on his face. "Because of a rise in Global temperature, there is a direct correlation to lower productivity seen in the lake. Southern winds create up wells of deep nutrient – rich water on the southern end of the lake. This happens during the cooler months of May to September. These nutrients that are in deep water are vital in maintaining the aquatic food chain. Global warming is slowing down the Southern winds there by limiting the ability for the mixing of nutrients."

"Are you a Marine Biologist?" Marx asked amused by Mr.Simfukwe's knowledge about the lake.

"You could call me that. I have lived for nearly fifty years by the shores of this lake. My fore- fathers fished in this lake," he explained taking a deep breath of the cool breeze that swept across to where they stood. "My hobbies include swimming, diving in Lake Tanganyika, Fishing and gathering information about this lake."

"You are definitely an expert on the lake," said Marx parting Mr. Simfukwe on the back.

"I see you are interested too, let me tell you more about Global warming and its devastating effects on Lake Tanganyika," Mr. Simfukwe continued encouraged by his curious student. "A research by O'Reilly and colleagues provides the strongest link to date between long – term changes in lake warming in the tropics, recorded by instruments and declining productivity of the lake's ecosystem as seen in sediment cores. Their work provided a clear indication of the regional effects of global climate and especially global warming on tropical lake ecosystems and in particular that of Lake Tanganyika. Continued climate warming has some severe implication for the nutrition and economy of the region's people who depend heavily on the lake. Those temperature changes stabilize the water column in lakes, especially in the tropics where, unlike in temperate regions, winter cooling and mixing is absent. The increased stability, decreased circulation, hampers the re- supply of nutrients from the deep water to the surface waters of the lake where they help algae grow. The algae, which form the base of Lake Tanganyika food chain, ultimately feed the commercially important fish, such as *Mpulungu Kapenta.* The fish population is starving and is reducing rapidly. Fishermen see this as a reduced catch in their nets. As a result, the famous and endemic Tanganyika sardines is now scarce on the market and becoming infamously expensive. In the past 80 years, fish stocks have reduced by 30% in Lake Tanganyika. Algae abundance declined by 20% in the same period. This was due to a reduction in lake circulation."

Dr Marximillian walked around Mpulungu port pleased to have met a self educated Marine Biologist. Across the Lake, he admired the green bushes on the mountains in the distance.

"What are the names of those mountains over there?" he asked walking over to where their tour guide stood chatting with the chief's daughter.

A range of hills formed a boundary in the distance, 200 meters from where they stood. Another blue mountain range could be seen farther away in the distance.

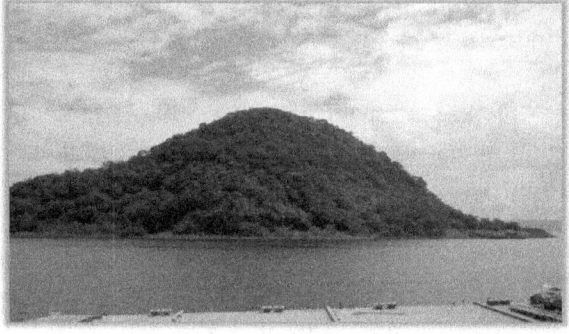

"To us the Lungu people of these lands, those aren't mountains, *Mipashi.* They are ancestral spirits. That one across is called Mbita and next to Mbita, is Namukale. Mpulungu is this one to our left,"

"What is the name of that blue mountain beyond Namukale? I like blue mountains," the chief's daughter asked pointing to a range of Blue Mountains on their left, in the space between Namukale and Mpulungu.

"That is Kapembwa. It looks blue because it is very far away," the Marine Biologist answered. "The island over there is Crocodile Island."

"I can see houses. Do people live there? Is that a fish camp?" Marx asked pointing to an island west of Mbita.

"People have settled on that Island. They live there," the guide explained.

Several large cranes hovered above their heads. The guide noticed Marx looking at the cranes curiously.

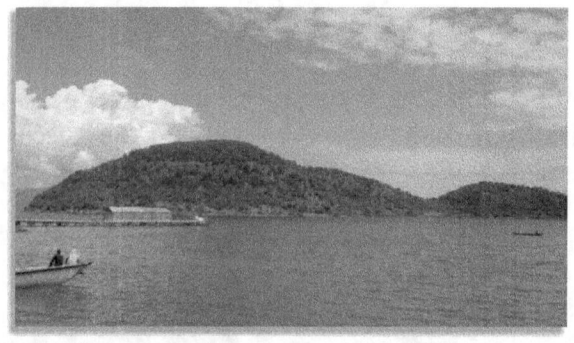

"This black and yellow crane over there is a 60,000 tone machine. It can lift a locomotive train," he explained.

Marx and the Chief's daughter thanked their guide and left Mpulungu Harbor overjoyed.

"Incredible lake; approximate length 700 km, that's like the distance from Livingstone to Kabwe," Marx remarked opening the door for his princess.

"Depth, approximately 1,500 meters and width 72 km," she added tapping on the dash board and raised her feet with excitement. "What would you like us to check out next?"

"Let us check out the fish market by the lake," he suggested.

"I was expecting to hear Kalambo falls. Do you want to buy fish at the Lake?" she asked smiling. "The Kalambo Falls is the second deepest uninterrupted single water falls in Africa. It is about 220m deep. It is deeper than the Mighty Victoria falls, which are the world's largest waterfalls. We should go there some time, you will love it."

They drove to the market discussing the amazing Lake Tanganyika.

***

They found a boat Ambulance on the shore. It had brought a patient from a rural health centre located on the lake. A pleasant community health assistant was the captain of this emergency rescue Marine Ambulance. He was delighted to meet Marx and the Princess. He offered to take them for a two hour trip on the lake.

His ambulance was a basic wooden boat powered by a small petrol engine. On this boat, it took an hour to reach his post. He told Marx he had brought a patient to Mpulungu hospital. She was pregnant and had been convulsing. Marx made a diagnosis of eclampsia. He turned to his princess and remarked.

"Imagine being on this boat with a woman convulsing on you,"

"Just the waves alone are tossing us like this, I bet it is a very dangerous and risk operation. They need a bigger modern boat," she suggested.

"Worse when you have to evacuate a convulsing patient in the middle of the night. There are about Ten million people who inhabit Lake Tanganyika watershed with an estimated growth rate of 2-3% per year," the captain explained steering his boat to the left towards some beautiful hills. "The highest population density is in Burundi at 250 persons per square kilometer. Zambia has the lowest number inhabiting the Tanganyika watershed. Guess how many?"

Marx was running his fingers on the blue water in the lake. The Princess was busy taking photos of him. They were enjoying the cool breeze on the lake.

"I think 10 persons per square kilometer," the princes answered laughing.

"Not bad, it is 13persons per square kilometer," the captain said laughing.

"Wow that is equivalent to each one of them owning eight football pitches or eight hectors," Isabelle quick brain computed an analogy.

"You would make the best Social worker of this water shed," said Marx looking at his Princess.

"I wonder how much fish is caught annually from this lake," she commented taking a picture of Marx.

"The annual fish catch from Lake Tanganyika is approximately 200,000 tonnes, with clupeids accounting for 65% of this catch," Their eyes met, this time she did not drop her gaze.

"I guess Mpulungu Kapenta is an example of Clupeids," she suggested.

"That's very true. They are known as Limnothrissa Miodon or commonly, Lake Tanganyika Sardine and locally simply called Mpulungu Kapenta. Whereas Lumpu in Burundi and dagaa in Tanzania," he explained beaming with excitement.

"Dagaa popa is different from our Kapenta," the captain corrected Marx. "Many simply call them Tu-dagaa. They have a notorious dorsal fin that must be removed before cooking."

"You are right, Dagaa is Rastrineobola argentea. Our Mpulungu Kapenta makes up the major biomass of fish in this lake. It is a planktivorous fresh water clupeid. What do you call a group of Mpulungu Kapenta?" he explained and asked his smart princess.

"It is known as a school," she smiled. "How come you know so much about fish? Have you ever heard about imbowa?"

"Yes, I am a fisherman too," he smiled and thought about Ms Isaacs. He had told her he was a fisherman on their long bus ride to Mbala. He wondered whether she would equal the intelligence of his Mpulungu Princess.

"You are thinking about someone," she remarked with a searching look at his face.

"You caught me ready 'minded'. How did you know? I was thinking about you eating imbowa," he lied. "Imbowa is 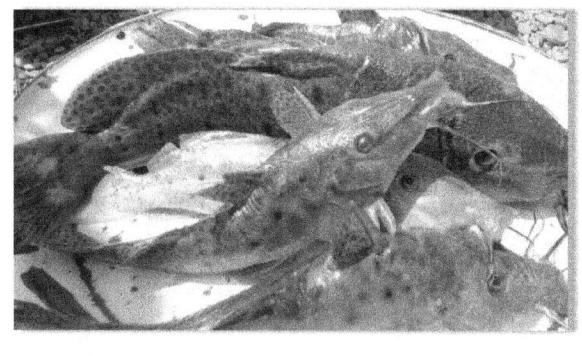 Auchenoglanis Occidentalis Tanganicanus or more commonly, Tanganyikan Giraffe Catfish. It is a Catfish. Both Prof P K Chishala and Don Williams sung about Catfish. I bet these fishes are truly tasty. This is a very gender sensitive fish. Only Males dig and make nests. The males tend the brood. Females scatter Eggs in a nest were they are guarded by the males. These African Catfish eat plants off the floor of lakes and streams. They belong to the kingdom Animalia and phylum Chordata. Some people love to keep this Catfish in aquariums. They are highly adaptable fish. They can accept a variety of food and tolerate a wide variety of water conditions.

"Really, and what else did you think about me?" she asked while taking photos of the beautiful spirit mountains in the distance.

"You are not wearing a life vest. Thought of how I would jump in the water to rescue you if this ambulance capsized," he explained and smiled.

She laughed and moved to sit next to him. The captain watched his two passengers curiously. He decided to stay out of their conversation and let them enjoy each other's company. He had no doubts in his mind; the princes deeply admired this man she was with.

He waited curiously to witness Marx pull out a small blue box and pop out a diamond ring. And kneel on the ambulance wet floor with the princess' hand in his and utter the words...generation of men have fooled women with, "Will you marry me". Fortunately, the trick still worked today.

The captain took his boat further on the lake to the Spirit Mountains. He was trying to aid his comrade by creating a perfect moment for two souls to connect. A chemical reaction was in progress and just needed a little catalyst to speed up things.

"That's Mbita, Namukale, Mpulungu and Kapembwa," she pointed out the Spirit Mountains. They were passing very close to Mbita.

The captain watched his love birds amuse themselves with the beautiful scenery on the lake. However, the ring was not coming out.

There was so much to see and photograph. Marx wished he had been trained in SCUBA diving. He would have taken his princess to watch the Gender sensitive fishes making nests at the bottom of the lake.

"Owing to their good parenting habits, the Giraffe Catfish are often abused by a related fish but from a different family and genus; Dinotopterus Cunningtoni. The Cunningtoni, take advantage of the giraffe

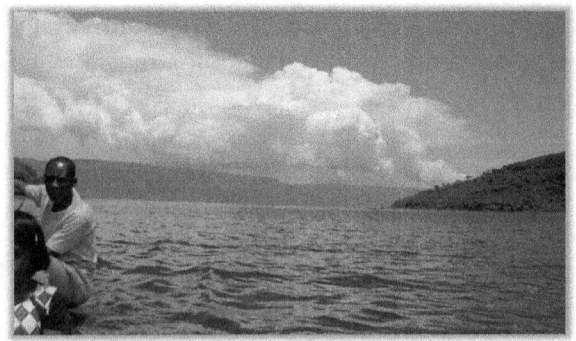

Catfish and allows the male to care for its eggs and young. This is an example of inter species brood care. Whereas the Giraffe catfish can only reach 30 cm in length, its cousin, the Cunningtoni grows up to 175 cm in length. It is large enough to feed two large families for a month," Marx continued his Catfish story.

The captain was disappointed with him seeing the anticipated diamond ring wasn't popping out from his breast pocket. He was splashing water with his left hand in the lake as he talked about catfish instead of presenting the diamond ring. The princess looked very beautiful against the billion stars sparkling in the water and the blue sky above. The captain felt like throwing Marx over board for failing to respond to the enchanting spirit mountains' beckoning call to propose.

The water sparkled in the sunlight above and gave a radiant blue color. The lake looked deceitfully calm. However Marx knew, if they capsized here, it would be a kilometer plunge into the Abyss. They had no life vests on. He was afraid to weigh the prospects of saving himself or his princess. He feared she would drag him to the bottom.

"Do you know how to swim?" he asked her.

"Don't worry I wouldn't jump on your back if we capsized. Instead I would race you to shore, if you knew how to swim that is," she laughed taking his hand in hers. "I am feeling cold."

A gentle cool breeze blew across the Lake. Crystal clear blue waves beat against the ambulance haul. They tossed their small wooden boat from side to side. There were several fishing boats on the lake and several local passenger boats.

The captain turned his wooden boat at the far end of Namukale feeling deeply disappointed and headed for the shore. Marx had a pleasant time on the water. The chief's daughter rested her head on Marx's left shoulder and wrapped her hands around his left arm. She was tired. She had worked all night at the hospital the previous day. Her incredibly warm body was synchronized with the waves and melodically bumped into Marx's huge muscular flank. He allowed himself to be tossed along like a pendulum. He admired the princess immensely. He stroked her long black hair. He thought 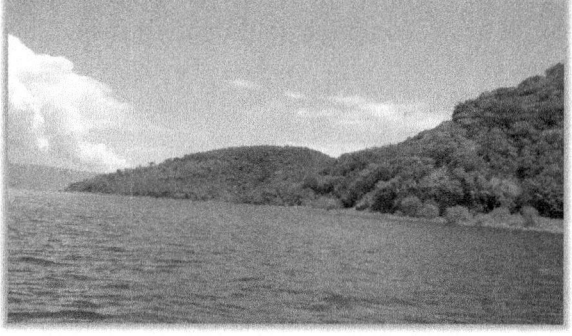 she was very beautiful and vulnerable. He vowed never to take advantage of her. He would protect her from the selfish desires of his flesh brewing inside his body at that hour.

When they reached the shore, he carried her from the boat and waded carefully to reach dry land. She curled herself and held tightly to his strong neck. She buried her head on his chest enjoying his masculine scent. He could hear her heart beating fast under the influence of his pheromones. A sweet acetone breath attended her exhaled air. Marx gave her a working diagnosis of Multi Orifice Starvation Syndrome, *MOSS*. He placed her on dry ground but remained wrapped around his neck. The local fishermen and traders watched Marx and Isabelle curiously. The locals were deeply *Marximesmerized.*

Marx thanked the captain and drove off with his princess to see another historical site. By now, it was 2 pm.

***

The oldest stone church in Zambia is found in Mpulungu. Marx and the Princess drove up hill on a tarred road to reach the site. The view of the lake below was spectacular. The worshipers at this historical church must have felt they were in heaven.

"Wow, would you look at that?" the Chief's daughter remarked.

"It is beyond my imagination. I was expecting to find only a foundation," said Marx walking towards the entrance of a giant tower at the front. He couldn't wait to get inside.

However, what he found horrified him. He was halted at the entrance by a reek of an obnoxious odor. He quickly turned round to prevent Isabelle from seeing the abomination inside the holy church.

"We can't go in there," he said.

"Why?" Isabelle the chief's daughter asked puzzled.

"It has been desecrated. People have turned it into a toilet. It smells awful inside there," bemoaned Marx.

Dr Marximillian was deeply hurt by the vandalism and neglect of this iconic structure. His lively chatter was suddenly put on mute. He stood in silence looking at the stone structure. It stood on open ground without a fence to keep out vandals. The trees around the church did not have tags indicating their names. Marx identified several Miombo trees and some

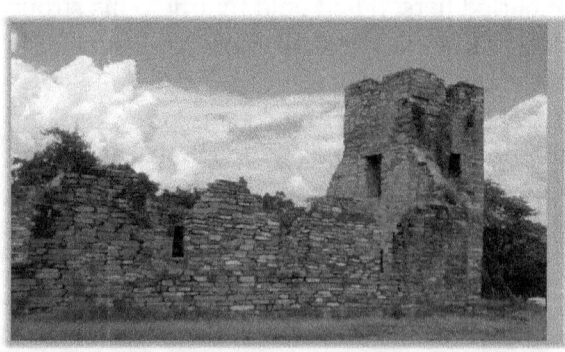

Umungamununsi. In the bushes behind the old church, he identified several Acacia Albina, Isoberlia Angolensis, Vitex Doniana and Galcinia species.

There was no curator or information office on site. Marx wished he could be appointed curator of this holy site. His astronomical mind would revolutionize the site and make it extremely attractive to tourists like Stonehenge in Wiltshire or the ivory-white marble mausoleum, the Taj Mahal.

"These fools have desecrated Niamkolo Church," he remarked angrily.

Isabelle walked over to him and wrapped her hands around his left arm.

"Don't be angry," she said. "Someone gets paid to care for this site. This is a clear sign; taxpayer's money is being stolen. There are people out there, whose job it is to look after such gazetted sites."

"I really wanted to see the interior of the church," he complained.

After suffering a resounding disappointment, Marx and Isabelle resigned themselves to enjoying the view of the Spirit Mountains and Lake Tanganyika Archipelago from this historical vintage point, Niamkolo Highlands. Had Dr David Livingstone stood here, he would have remarked, "After twenty minutes sail from Lake Tanganyika and a short drive up hill, we came in sight, for the first time, ancient columns of brick walls, appropriately called Niamkolo church. It had never been seen before by a few good doctors' eyes; but scenes so lovely must have been gazed upon by angels in their flight."

"Tell me about your ex," she said changing the subject and clung to his big left arm.

"No, it is a sad story," he answered stroking her hands with his right palm.

"Please," she pleaded with him.

"It is a very bad story. I really don't think you should hear it. It will make you very sad," he said. "I don't want to see your beautiful face turn red on me."

"Actually, I would be very sad if you didn't tell me," she said pulling on his arm.

"Don't say I didn't warn you," he started. "We were married for seven years then she divorced me,"

"Divorced you, why?" she asked concerned.

"She came home one Friday night drunk, this was after disappearing from home for a week. When I asked where she had been, she told me to cut off her head and get the answer from her throat," he said.

"Why was she tempting you into committing such a hideous crime? She is lucky it was you, a compassionate and civilized man," she remarked thoughtfully. "Had it been a barbaric man, he would have sliced her throat open or shot her or stabbed her to death and then killed himself. She should thank you for sparing her life."

"For the first time in my life; in a brief yet protracted moment, I wrestled thoughts men who kill face. Irresistible dark feelings coaxed me and dragged me towards a slippery Zero Option cliff," he explained recalling the agonizing anger that had consumed him.

"You are a great man, you walked away from a crime many weak men wouldn't have; Men who beat or kill react in split seconds and slay their wives like vicious senseless beasts. They are consumed by intense emotions of anger, incapacitating them from rational thinking and slip off the cliff you stood steadfast on and restrained your hand from being stained with filthy blood whoring around. These men are like wounded beasts whose sole purpose is to devour their spouses or girlfriends they perceive to be cheating on them," she lectured him.

"I think she was expecting me to react that way because when she returned home that heinous night, she looked extremely terrified. She sat on the bed in the spare bedroom and curled herself in the corner trembling. She screamed and hurled insults using the most horrendous and diabolical foul language I have ever heard come out of a human mouth. To think I ever kissed that mouth made me sick and had to go to the bathroom to throw up," he explained. "Until that day, I knew her as my little angel of nine years."

"What was making her behave with such impropriety, indecency, immorality, shameless rudeness and vulgarity?" she asked in disbelief.

"I really don't know. To my knowledge, this was the first time she had ever disappeared from home. It was the first time she had ever exhibited this outlandish behavior," he told the story recalling the night he stood in the spare

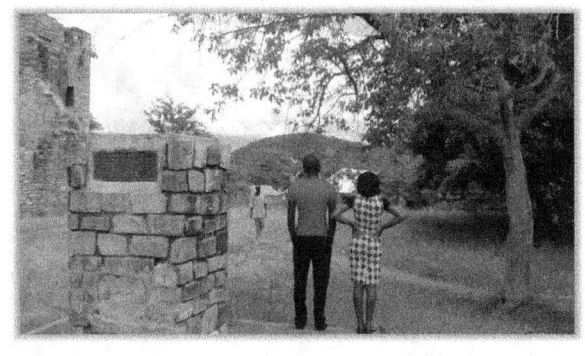

room of his house at 3am bewildered by his estranged wife's behavior. "She refused to leave the spare room. Her eyes burnt deeply red as she hurled these obscenities at me. I decided to leave her alone hoping she would come back to her senses,"

"It must have been hard on the children having a whoring mom," she said deeply affected by Marx's tale. "Did she leave the spare room?"

"She lived alone in this room, like a giant nocturnal creature, for the next one month while I stayed in the main bedroom with my boys. I expected her to calm down, and come out of her acute psychotic state. At the beginning of the second month, she came home one evening with summons to court for divorce," he told Isabelle.

"What! And she still hadn't explained where she had disappeared to," Isabelle exclaimed.

"Not without decapitation, she wouldn't tell me anything," he explained.

"What did you do?" she asked wiping a tear from her eye.

"I consulted a very senior officer in the province who was in charge of my department. This was an incredibly wise man. He was retiring that year after an illustrious long career in management. I was shocked by what he told me; his exact words were; 'Doc, I don't want to buy you a Coffin. I am transferring you with immediate effect. If you spend just one more night in your house, you will die....I am glad you came just in time; Information has reached this office; don't ask me how or why... there are powerful and evil people who want to take over your home,' he didn't mince his words. I was speechless,"

"Cold blooded murderous bastards; they wanted to kill you over a woman... I bet she must have been a very pretty girl," she laughed. "She was an attractive *She-Devil,* wasn't she?"

"You see, you are laughing at me," he smiled. "You are right; she was a very beautiful young lady, a descendant of a legendary breed of beautiful women born on the plains of central Africa following the Zulu wars of southern Africa. I was proud of her. She made me look handsome. She was my best friend for nine years. We were a very happy family,"

"Honestly, what went wrong? What happened? I think you should have gone ahead and cut her throat open," she giggled.

"Do you know who a She Devil is?" he asked

"I think I do; it is your friend's recent ex-wife; a temptress who has an amazing influence on men; she can ensnare you to commit any act she bequests regardless of your foundation. The devil is kind compared to her. If you visit her you will want to keep your shoes on," she explained smiling.

"That is correct, a She Devil is a woman who resembles the devil, as in extreme wickedness, cruelty, or bad temper," he reiterated Isabelle's definition. "My ex's sudden behavior change can only be explained by a fellow woman. It couldn't be explained by a man, not even by a Psychiatrist or Priest. She had been promised a job in the diplomatic service."

"What! Forgive me for saying this; I think she was a senseless restless *She-Devil Bitch.* How could a sane woman with beautiful children, agree to a plot to kill her selfless hard working husband just over some damn Foreign Service job?" she exclaimed staring down at the spirit mountains from Niamkolo Highlands.

"Anyhow, after the wise counsel from my director, I went back to my house to pack a small bag. I got my laptop and fled town with only the cloths I wore," he explained admiring Lake Tanganyika and the spirit mountains in the distance.

"Did you find out who these people were?" she asked curiously.

"He was afraid to name them. I could only suspect," he answered.

"What did she do when you left?" she probed further.

"She sued for divorce, alleging that I had abandoned the family. In court, an idiot called me a criminal in a parked open court room,"

"Why didn't you tell the court your life was in danger?"

"I couldn't; I didn't have any evidence to back my claims and I couldn't bring my director to testify. I would have put his life in danger too. She had risen above discipline," he explained. "She sued several other senior people during the same period over silly matters; even over coughing and laughing."

"I think I have an idea at just the sort of wicked people that would confer such defiant stupidity on a bitch like that," Isabelle drew her conclusion admiring the Spirit Mountains in the distance.

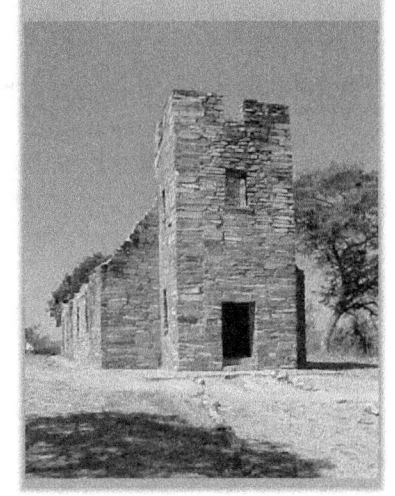

"More recently, nearly three years today, she sued me again in another court, demanding more money from me. This time, I faced a midget, a fellow whose Judgment was clearly riddled with a reek of prejudice. He had been raised by a single mom and saw in me his father's escapades. He hated his father with all his heart. I found out his father had walked out on his mother when he was little. All the anger he had harbored against his own father, he unleashed it on me. He called me a criminal and even threatened to throw me into jail,"

"That is a shame. I have never heard of a criminal who works as hard as you do and one who is as compassionate as you. If criminals looked like you, then I love criminals," she said in disbelief.

"The day before I travelled here, I was again in court. She was demanding for more money," he narrated his recent ordeal walking towards Niamkolo church. "The court took away my salary... This is how I ended up here, trying to make ends meet. Sometimes, I pray these evil people should die a painful slow death, even when I know that I ought to pray for my enemies who plot to hurt me. I know vengeance is for the LORD; however I feel like avenging them myself. I want them to die painful slow deaths for doing this to me. However, I know I must forgive them."

"What about the children?" she asked. "You should bring them I look after them. I love children very much."

"The court put a restraining order. I can't see my children. She even threatened to change their names. I think she did," he said.

"What? Unless you are not their Father," she remarked. "You lived with the most evil person I have ever heard about."

"I told myself, unless my blood does not flow in the veins of those boys; it will flow back home whatever the court decision. Nothing can stand in its way. Blood is thicker than water," he explained smiling at Isabelle who now had her small arms around Marx's waist. "I have never told this story to anyone. Forgive me for dragging you into my troubles."

"A problem shared, is a problem solved. Thank you for trusting me with your story. I didn't know we had such evil women in our country. Allow me to ease the pain of your aching heart. I think your ex- was possessed by a dog spirit. She cannot be satisfied by a legion of adulterous men. She roams the streets like a bitch on heat. She lurks around streets corners looking for someone to mount her. All disgusting bodily fluids discharged by the adulterous into her bottomless whoring pit can't fill it nor satisfy her. She tries to find ways to harm you by taking your children hostage. However, soon the children will grow up and leave her. She must seek deliverance or she will die on the streets like a homeless dog on Heat," Isabelle consoled Marx. "What do you call it in science?"

"Estrous," Marx answered thoughtfully. "It is the time in a bitch's cycle when she displays intense interest in mating. Estrous begins when the bitch allows the male to mount her and ends when her receptive behavior ceases. I think in women possessed by the dog Spirit in Estrous, this pervasive whoring behavior does not cease." He recalled his disobedience to the almighty when he took this bitch as his unlawfully wedded wife. He deeply regretted his actions on this hot Mpulungu afternoon.

Marx and Isabelle stood in each other's arms admiring the landscape all around them. Niamkolo Highlands offered an incredible panoramic view of the Spirit Mountains and Lake Tanganyikan archipelago.

The church Dr Marximillian was crying over was built by the London Mission Society from 1893 – 1896. It is the oldest surviving stone built church in Zambia. A fifteen meter tower that has survived to this very day forms the façade of the building. This three storey tower served as a light house to boats on the lake below. The main hall of the church is made of one meter thick walls. The Niamkolo Church was declared a National Monument in April 1955.

The blend of colours all around them fascinated Dr Marximillian; the vegetation; trees and the grass were a deep green colour. The Spirit Mountains, Mbita and Namukale, covered by a canopy of green bushes, 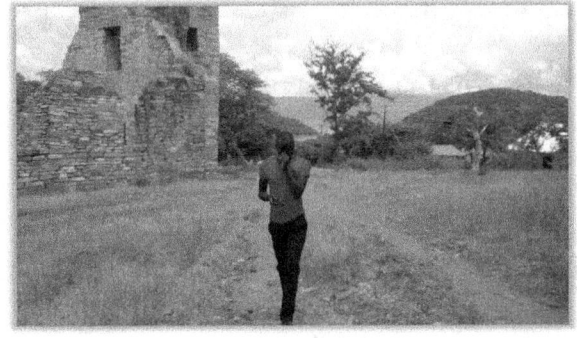 could be seen towering above the blue lake below. Further away, the Sky Blue Spirit Mountain could be seen stretching across and blend with the blue sky above. White clouds stretched across in the distance above Kapembwa like a thick coat of paint from a painter's brush. Niamkolo church blended beautifully against this background. The elements of time had turned its stone walls into a golden grayish brown colour. Marx was certain, if this had been a painting, it would be a priceless master piece.

***

Dr Marximillian returned from Mpulungu rejuvenated. The following day, Monday, was very busy at the hospital.

A Stitch in Time

T his was Marx's second week in Mbala. He lay on his bed reminiscing the wonderful time he had in Mpulungu with the Chief's daughter the previous day.

He eagerly looked forward for things to easy up and to a great day at work. The driver was late to pick him. He decided to pass the time watching international news. American politics dominated all news channels. The republican leading candidate Donald Trump had just lost in Wisconsin to Ted Cruz. A news headline raced across the wide plasma screen; 'Cruz Victory throws Republic race into Turmoil,' it read.

Dr Marximillian studied this news bulletin curiously.

While he was thinking, a beautiful reporter appeared on the screen. 'Sanders gains momentum after Wisconsin win,' she said.

"Bernie Sanders needs huge wins to catch Clinton," another commented.

The American presidential race had just become exciting. Marx admired the resilience demonstrated by the candidates. While the winners celebrated their short lived victories, the losing candidates gracefully accepted their loss and were already looking forward to the next stop in the race. They did not sit back and mourn over their losses. Marx realized, losing was another form of winning. He was not going to allow loss of pay hinder him from winning elsewhere.

He took a Taxi to hospital after waiting in vain for his hospital transport. It was raining outside.

He rushed to male surgical ward to see Moses, his cholecystostomy patient. This was his most complicated case since arriving at ACH.

Now he was sure, he had outlived his welcome. Broke as he was, he was subsidizing the institution's transport cost.

Moses was delighted to see Dr Marximillian. He leaped from his bed to meet Marx and showed him his drain. He was eating his regular meals now. The wound was healing well.

"Uli Moses?" Dr Marximillian greeted him.

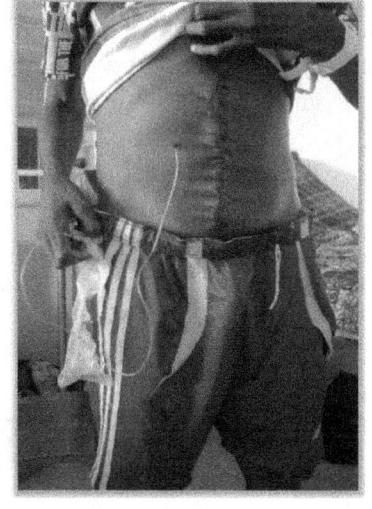

"Ningo sili, ya doctor," he answered.

"How is the wound?" he asked.

"Chikuwaya panono," he answered.

"I was on Lake Tanganyika yesterday," said Marx studying his patient's face carefully.

"Really, I miss home," said Moses looking down. "That lake is my home and my work place. I am a fisherman. Now I don't know if I will be able to catch fish again. It is the only Job I know."

"I will discharge you today. I want you to go home. Take walks to Mpulungu harbor and enjoy the view of the lake from Niamkolo Church. This will accelerate your healing. Then in six to eight weeks, come back to the hospital and we will remove this tube," Marx told his patient.

"Really, I would be very delighted; do you eat Kapenta Ya Doctor? I will bring you a bag of Kapenta and Fresh fish when I come for my review. Thank you for saving my life. I would have died and been forgotten by now. I should find you when I come," Moses made promises excited to be going home to Lake Tanganyika.

Marx was delighted. He was happy his trip to Mbala had not been in vain. His surgical skills had just saved a life. If his persecutory journey up north had been worth anything, it was Moses. He was convinced if he had to travel to attend just one person, like Moses, he would make it over and over again. He was sad he would not be around to see Moses when he came for review. He prayed God would send another competent doctor to ACH and attend Moses. The country needed many skills like those Marx was endowed with.

Unfortunately, those entrusted with sourcing these skills and harnessing them locally didn't think so. They didn't care a bit about people like Dr Marximillian. Marx wished his skills were transferable like a piece of garment; he would have simply passed it to another to wear while he slipped off into oblivion. He had the wisdom to know, he was not indispensable as an individual, however his skills were. The country could not run without health care professionals. Many vulnerable citizens would die, particularly women and children.

The country was in dire need of people like Marx. Dr Mukonka Chiti had been let down by incompetent Human Positioning Scouts. He was convinced *The System* needed an overhaul. It had been infiltrated by too many rotten eggs and corrupt square pegs.

It needed strict tools to monitor and evaluate its performance. Dr Chiti felt a tool to measure the rate at which essential skills where being lost in the country needed to be devised. The country could not go on losing skills and be turned into a dwelling for fools.

As he left the ward, he thought of teachers like Daliso who were under performing at various schools they taught owing to the burden of debt and other hardships facing them. When the country borrows senselessly, the citizens suffered from the carelessness of those entrusted with the management of the country's economy. Similarly, when the citizens borrowed senselessly or thrust into financial despondency as was Dr Marximillian and Mr. Daliso Banda, it was the country that suffered ultimately. Absenteeism from work, underperformance, skills loss, theft at work, slowed spending, mass unemployment; all would impact negatively on economical growth. It is the duty of the state to protect its entire citizenry from sliding down this path, particularly essential workers as their skills took a life time for a nation to nurture.

The cheap Chinese doctors Misdirector and Misdirected planned to replace Marx with took the honourable Chinese Government a hundred years to foster. The foolish scouts at Marx's position filing resources where planning to harvest were they did not sow.

The Financial Symbiosis of State revenue or borrowing and expenditure on one hand; Citizens borrowing, skills driven wages or salaries and expenditure on the other, must be kept in a state of rotatory equilibrium to generate energy and power national development. This was Marx's first principle of Rotatory Economics.

***

After a light lunch in the hospital cafeteria, Marx hurried to Gynecology ward to see Rhoda. She had not received blood and her condition was now desperate. The student doctors, Jessy, Joan and Selym had joined him for lunch.

They followed him to learn how to manage severe anemia in a rural community hospital. They were met by Dr Kalunda in the wide corridor leading to the children's ward.

"You girls don't want to see me nowadays because of Dr Marximillian," he teased the medical students and stopped to greet Marx.

"How can we come to see you when you don't buy us lunch," Selym answered giggling.

"We just had a wonderful Lunch with Dr Marximillian," said Joan laughing.

"I can see you are fascinated working with Dr Marximillian," Dr Kalunda remarked. "He was my teacher too you know."

"I think they are *Marximused* if not *Marximesmerized*," said Marx laughing.

"I think they are *Marxihypnotized*," Kalunda answered smiling.

Just then, an Ambulance from the district office veered in. They all turned to see what it had brought. A nurse and another person emerged shortly aiding a patient who could hardly stand. Marx quick mind noticed the patient could not support her own head. She was dragging her feet between the shoulders rushing her to Maternity.

"Doc, that patient is in shock," said Marx rushing to check on the patient. "Put her down. Lay her on the floor."

The nurse and her assistance put the patient down wondering what was going on.

"We are rushing her to Maternity," the nurse answered after placing the patient down.

"No, you are rushing her to her death," Marx snapped at the poor nurse.

Meanwhile Dr Kalunda was kneeling by the body on the floor checking for pulses. She had no running Intravenous Access.

"Which health post are you from?" he asked.

"The patient is suffering from anemia in pregnancy. She came to our centre last night. She was just ok," the poor nurse answered.

"I think she is just hungry," the nurse's assistance answered.

"And who are you?" Marx asked him.

"I am the community health assistance," he answered proudly looking at Marx.

"You were right doc, this woman is in shock. All her peripheries are cold. Unfortunately, we don't have blood in the hospital," Dr Kalunda explained with audible quiver in his voice.

Marx bent down and examined the patient. He rose immediately, "This woman has a ruptured uterus. Dr Joan, rush bring two gray Cannulars from the ward, Dr Jessica bring surgical gloves and two litters saline, Ka Selym bring a stretcher," Marx gave clear military orders to his assiduous doctors.

By now, this make shift Corridor Emergency Room had attracted several other student doctors; Agnes, Sipho, Natasha, Esther and Kaluba gathered eager to lend a hand.

"Doctors, we are at DEFCON 2," he explained the situation to the new arrivals.

"Defcon; is she dead?" Esther asked wondering what Dr Marximillian meant by DEFCON 2.

"The Defense Readiness Condition, DEFCON, is an alert state used by the United States Military. We could call ours ERCON; for Emergency Readiness Condition but I like the sound of DEFCON," Marx explained.

Johnny Mbala arrived pushing a trolley with Ka Selym. Sr Agnes Francis was a beautiful student Nun, always calm and collected. She arrived carrying specimen bottles to collect samples for the laboratory. O'Neil appeared at the corridor emergency room holding a urine bag. Dr Marximillian sent Kaluba and Felix Katongo to inform theatre staff to prepare to receive a very sick woman and to set the theatre alertness to DEFCON 2.

"Shouldn't we first take her to Maternity?" Johnny Mbala asked.

"My dear Dr Johnny this is war. We are at DEFCON 2; we are going straight to theatre from here. We are ready to engage the threat. We can't afford to waste another hour, we could lose this patient. This is not DEFCON 5 where you have lowest state of readiness" he answered. "Sr Francis, go to the blood bank. Tell them Dr Marximillian Mukonka Chiti wants five collecting bags for blood *IMMEDIATELY*."

Now, Johnny had a long bearded chin that gave him an exceptionally pious look. He was an unusually quiet fellow with a keen eye. He had wanted to become a priest but the desires of his flesh prevented him. He found he was not cut out for a long lonely life of celibacy. There was rumour among his fellow students that he had run away from a Tibetan Monastery. He loved Sr Francis a great deal and often teased her. She invoked memories in him that conspired against the prospective Father Johnny, and probably a future pope.

"Are you planning on conducting auto transfusion?" Dr Kalunda asked. "I am coming to see. I have never seen this being done."

"Most certainly; there are four litters of free blood inside her belly. I am not planning on wasting it," Dr Marximillian answered beaming with excitement on his face.

Joan's saline bottles were, by now, running down the patient's veins. Torrents of rain had not let off since morning. The exotic trees that adorned the façade of Abercorn Community Hospital swayed beautifully in the Rain. Collection of drizzles from the roof ran down the drainage on the edge of the corridor like an agitated shallow seasonal stream. A haze could be seen over the surrounding areas. Old Location, Kampompo and new Location Townships were covered in thick fog. It was freezing outside. This was the weather that had attracted the white settlers to Abercorn. With average annual temperature of 18.7 degrees, Mbala was truly a seat of London weather.

***

Marx and his team arrived in theatre. They put their patient on supplemental oxygen and continued to stabilize her for surgery. The theatre nurse was busy arranging her instruments on the operating table.

Dr Marximillian ran through the steps for auto transfusion. He told his students what they were about to witness was not standard practice. He told them, in Africa; desperate situations called for desperate solutions at the front lines of Emergency Rural Health Care Delivery.

"Emergency Health Care in Rural Africa is not different from care during armed conflict or war," he explained. "The blood we are about to use has many impurities. It is mixed with amniotic fluid, Vernix Caseosa and possibly meconium. She may even have Vernix Caseosa Peritonitis, a rare but serious complication seen following Caesarean section. It is thought to occur as a result of spillage of amniotic fluid and or meconium into the maternal peritoneal cavity. Uterine rapture in our patient has done exactly that."

"What is Vernix Caseosa?" Joan asked.

"Is the waxy or cheese-like white substance found coating the skin of newborn human babies," he answered.

"How does Vernix Caseosa peritonitis start," Johnny Mbala asked.

"I will explain after the operation, you must remind me. I must scrub in now, our patient is ready. Joan and Jessica I will need you to stand next to me on my right but mind the sterile field. You will hold the filtering chamber for the blood. It will run down a giving set attached to it into a receiving bag. Felix and Kaluba will be holding the receiving bag or reinfusion bag. They will pass the collected pints of blood to Agnes and Johnny who will connect the bag to the line running into the patient's veins and pump the blood back into the patient's vascular compartment. Musonda, you will squeeze the pint of blood on the right and Kaoma, will squeeze the one on the left. Dr Kalunda, you will scrub in with me. You can wash and prep the patient's abdomen while I check whether these guys have got their roles well," he instructed his team calmly.

The anaesthetist was impressed with Dr Marximillian's sense of calm leadership in the face of an emergency. He gave the team confidence even when they were faced with a dire situation. Watching Marx in theatre was like working with a seasoned, battle tested Army commander.

"Dr Marx, won't that lead to Vernix Caseosa SIRS?" Agnes asked.

"SIRS; Systemic Inflammatory Response Syndrome, that is right Sr Francis," he answered.

"It is like Jumping out of the frying pan into the Fire," Father Johnny Mbala remarked. Every one burst out laughing.

"Jonny, do you know the meaning for your name?" Marx asked.

"No sir," he answered.

"It means one who has no fear; having courage; having a fine appearance. Gallant, courteous, like an ideal knight; someone with a special charm or allure that inspires allegiance or devotion; One of the, if not the coolest person you'll encounter in your life time. The most interesting man in the room at all times," he explained and everyone burst out laughing.

"OMG…no wonder I hear people say; *He's hung like Johnny!*" Joan remarked.

"I think the beard makes him the most interesting student in this theatre," Sr Francis teased him. "He looks like he jumped out of a frying pan himself."

"I am the coolest person you will ever encounter in your life time," he answered with a grin. "Doc, with no proper blood in the hospital this is definitely a frying pan-fire jumping desperado."

(Medical Jargon below [*in italics*], may skip without loss to story flow)

"You could call it that; only, in our situation, my dear Father Dr Johnny, the fire isn't burning yet. We may have a window of escape before the blaze engulfs the pan. In the case of Vernix Caseosa Peritonitis, it presents as an acute abdomen days to weeks after a seemingly uncomplicated caesarean section. Only a few cases have been reported to date. *The pathophysiology of VCP is incompletely understood. Histological examinations of biopsy specimens reveal anucleate squamous cells along with lanugo hair and foreign body giant cell reaction. The diagnosis must be considered in cases of post CS acute abdomen. Your question Sr Francis, this may be the first case of Vernix Caseosa Systemic Inflammatory Response Syndrome, VC-SIRS. It has never been reported in the literature. We are familiar with Amniotic Fluid embolism, a lethal killer.* We can only pray, our patient survives the fire," Dr Marximillian explained stepping on the operating table.

"Father Johnny will pray for her. She will just be alright," Sr Agnes remarked smirking at Johnny.

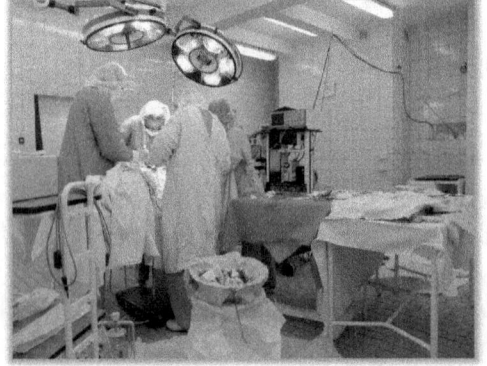

The nurse passed him the surgical knife. He made a short vertical incision below the patient's umbilicus. He dissected his way into the abdominal cavity carefully. There was no drop of blood to be found in the tissues of the abdomen. The patient was completely white. She had bled massively internally. A midwife had joined the team. She walked leisurely into theatre knowing the baby was dead.

"Doctor, there is no blood in the blood bank. They said the patient's hemoglobin was 7g/dl," she reported.

Marx did not answer her. By now, he had entered the peritoneal cavity. He asked the theatre nurse to pass him a Gallipot. The midwife rushed to turn on the suction machine upon seeing the sea of blood in the patient's abdomen.

"Switch off that machine," the anaesthetist ordered her.

"Dr Jessica and Dr Joan, are we ready? Dr Marximillian asked.

"We are ready sir," they answered.

He dipped the Gallipot inside the patient's abdomen and filled it with blood. He then poured it into the filter Jessica and Joan were holding. The deep dark red blood ran down a plastic tubing into the collecting bag Felix and Kaluba were holding. Soon one unit was ready for use. The priest connected it religiously and ran it down into the patient's veins.

"This looks like an Agricultural irrigation system or a Hydro-Engineering Science Model," Johnny observed.

"That's very true; the incision wound on the abdomen is like a well. The blood represents water. The Galipot is like a bucket for drawing water. And what Joan and Jessica are holding is like a reservoir tank," Ka Selym drew an analogy.

"This is an unconventional system you are observing. The actual system is elaborate; it has a collecting reservoir, like the one Joan is holding, which is connected to a vacuum. To the line of the shed blood is attached a bag containing an anticoagulant. The blood runs down a valve system and is mixed with a wash solution before entering the reinfusion bag such as the one Kaluba and Felix are holding," Marx explained to his mesmerized team.

The midwife was utterly Marximesmerized. She stood at the foot end of the operating table and watched in total bewilderment. By now, the team had collected five pints of blood.

Satisfied with the success of his ingenuity, Marx turned his attention to the dead baby in the womb. He grabbed it by the legs and passed it to the midwife still attached to the placenta at the umbilicus. It was covered with Vernix Caseosa.

"The waxy or cheese-like white substance coating the skin of the baby is Vernix Caseosa," Dr Marximillian explained holding the dead baby in his hands. "Joan, you can go and take a look."

He then turned his attentention to the uterus. It had suffered a wide posterior tear and could not be saved. There was no active bleeding from the edges. The tear extended from an old Caesar wound in front to the back and downwards to the vagina.

***

While Marx and Dr Kalunda worked frantically to remove the uterus, via an operation called total hysterectomy, the students chatted with the midwife in the neonatal resuscitation unit in the opposite room.

"The baby looks big, was it Mature?" Jessica asked.

"It is 3.5kg," the midwife answered after weighing it. "It was a girl."

"Where was she from? Why couldn't she go to the hospital early? She was a previous Caesar right," Joan asked looking sad.

"She was from Mpulungu," said Johnny

"An Island on lake Tanganyika," Ka Selym answered.

"Poor woman, maternal health services are very poor in that area," Felix remarked.

"Am sure she thought she could deliver at home," said Kaoma.

"She was afraid to go to hospital because of the previous caesarean she had. Many women don't go to hospital even when we advise them to," the midwife told the students.

"Why is it so?" Sipho asked. "Maybe you frighten them."

"They are usually afraid at the prospects of having another operation. I wouldn't be surprised to hear that this woman took traditional labour enhancing drugs," Johnny explained.

"Kaselelele, the traditional Oxytocin, that is most likely," the mid wife remarked. "Who is that new doctor you are with? I have never seen him. She must thank God for sending him here. This woman would have died."

"That's Dr Marximillian Mukonka Chiti," Joan answered rolling her eyes. "He is my hero."

While the students chatted with the midwife, Dr Marximillian had finished the operation. He washed the patient's abdomen copiously with saline to prevent VCP. He left two drains in the abdomen. He then asked Dr Kalunda to close the abdomen and scrubbed down.

He left the operating room and strode along the wide corridor stretching from the staff main entrance to the male change room on the eastern end. He was tired; it had been a long operation. He walked admiring the operating theatre at ACH deeply. It had several spacious rooms. The change rooms had showers. The duty room was spacious and had a television set for the staff and could be used as a conference room. Across, to where he stood, was another wide corridor stretching from the patient's main entrance. At the far end of this corridor, was a six bed recovery room. From here, a passage led to the maternity and labour ward. This passage was among the most important aqueducts in the hospital. His patient was due to use this passageway out of theatre. In all, there were three operating rooms inside this colossal theatre. These comprised two sterile operating rooms and a dirty cases operating area. In addition to operating room space, this theatre housed a large theatre supplies store room, operating sets and instruments room, a distiller and office space.

He stood for a while and stared out through the window on the eastern end of the operating theatre. The lawn outside between the gynaecology and surgical wards looked beautiful in the rain. He had forgotten, there was still a drizzle outside. It was now 5pm.

***

He left theatre to search for the unreliable hospital Wi-Fi signal. He wanted to check his mail. He was hoping to find an e-mail from Medicines San Frontieres or a hospital in Australia. He had resolved to join doctors without borders. He didn't mind prospects of deployment to a conflict zone. He had faced enough conflict in his country and paid a huge price. He was certain, somewhere far away, his skills would be respected and save a life.

There were several people outside when he left theatre. This was 5pm; it was the visiting hour at Abercorn Community Hospital.

***

Isabelle reported for work at 7pm, 2hrs after Marx had left theatre. She called him on her cell phone when she heard about the auto transfusion in theatre. Rumour and medical exploits travelled like wild fire at ACH. Everyone that heard was utterly Marximesmerized that a procedure like that could be done at ACH.

She was delighted to see him. It already felt like many months since she last saw him.

"You look beautiful Isabelle," he said reaching out to hug her.

"I missed you," she said. "I feel like I saw you more than a year ago, yet I was with you just yesterday."

They talked about Marx's patient, Auto transfusion, Mpulungu, Fish, Music, Movies, Love, Kalambo Falls, Chishimba Falls and the rain outside.

"Have you watched the Movie 'How High'? She asked him when they sat down.

"I love those crazy Harvard freshmen. They smoked their friend's ashes," said Marx laughing.

"How about, 'Like Heaven'? She asked.

"I think it is about a doctor who was in coma following a road traffic accident. And her ghost returned to her former apartment and tried to evict the new tenant," he answered.

"I like the way they fell in love," she said.

"He was a crazy chap; he fell in love with a ghost. He had issues with alcohol," Marx remarked laughing.

"Would you like to see my photos taken at Chishimba falls? But I must warn you, I was in a bikini," she asked getting her Samsung Tablet.

"Thou shall not lead me into temptation," he said taking the tablet from her hands.

"You can only be tempted if that was what you wanted all along," she burst out laughing. "I brought some supper, would you like to join me?"

"Wow, the food looks scrumptious. *Akatemba Cupo*," he remarked reaching out to taste.

"*Akatemba Cupo*. Who is teaching you proverbial Bemba? Do you know its meaning?" she asked studying his face carefully.

"Good cooking is the foundation of marital life," he answered smiling. "If you continue caring for me like this, I will shift to the palace and become the chief's advisor in law,"

"Time has moved very fast, I have to give medication now. Help me," she stood up to prepare the medicine trolley.

"Sometimes you start relationships, sometimes they start you," he murmured to himself.

"What? I can't get you. What are you saying?" she called from the medicine store room.

"I discharged Moses. I think he is in Mpulungu right now," he called out after her. "I kept only five patients for you on the ward. They are all on oral medication."

"You are so caring, thank you," she answered.

"Hey, can I leave you to work. I want to check on the post hysterectomy patient," he said standing to leave. He found Isabelle extremely vulnerable to his desires of the flesh. He had vowed never to take advantage of her. It was clear, she had *MOSS*.

She protested at his excuse to leave but soon obliged when he promised he would return.

***

At 11pm, Marx strode to Gynecology ward to see his patient. He found the nurses exhausted and resting in the duty room.

"How is the post Hysterectomy patient? How are her vitals?" he asked.

"That one, she is fine and even talking," the nurse answered pointing to a bed in the acute bay on the left. There were four critical patients in this bay. Marx called it the quadrangle of critical illness.

Rhoda, Marx's oldest patient lay on a bed direct opposite to were Dr Marximillian stood. She was frail. She was fading away. Her abdomen had distended again. An NG tube had been reinserted and was draining actively. She was dying. She was only 23.

There were two patients with peritonitis to Marx's immediate left, both had declined surgery. On Rhoda's immediate right, lay Marx's newest patient. She looked out of danger.

"Nurse, why are we nursing a post op patient sandwiched with peritonitis cases?" she will get infected and complicate into peritonitis too," Marx asked the nurse with disappointment in his voice.

"I was wondering too. She was placed here by the medical students. We thought that was what you wanted," the nurse answered.

"Come, let us move her out of here," said Marx walking towards his patient's bed.

"It is ok doctor, we will move her. You are tired, get some rest,"

Marx left the hospital after midnight. He was extremely tired. He could hardly keep his eyes open.

Round the Clock

H e awoke the next morning at six. He found a text from the chief's daughter sent at 3am. He decided to call her.

"You dozed on me," she protested.

"I am terribly sorry, I have just seen your text," he answered.

"I wanted to ask whether you would be in the hospital before 7am," she explained vaguely.

"Would you like me to see your patient?" he asked.

"I am the patient," she explained. "Can I wait for you?"

***

Dr Marximillian lay in bed wondering whether it was worth it continuing his work at the hospital. He looked at his traveler bag tacked away in one corner of his room. His services where no longer required at the ministry of Life. He decided he would leave as soon as he had discharged all the patients in his care.

In maternity, he found Rhoda's condition had deteriorated further. Her urine output had decreased to a critical level. Her legs were swollen and the intestines paralyzed. A feeding tube was draining a greenish fluid from her nose into a collecting back. Her husband stood by the bed side in disheveled cloths. He was a peasant Fisherman from Lake Tanganyika.

She covered herself in a blue chitenge from the waist downwards and supported her head on a pink pillow. She gazed at Dr Marximillian with searching eyes.

"Doctor, I sinned. I am being punished for my sin," she said when he came close to her bed.

"Don't talk like that Rhoda. We have all sinned. No one is without sin in the sight of God," Marx tried to comfort her. He took her hand in his. It felt very cold.

Rhoda's relatives approached Dr Marximillian to ask him whether they could take their patient away.

"Doctor, please allow me to take my daughter away," Rhoda's dad made a request.

"Her condition is critical sir. I wish I could do more to help save your daughter," He replied.

"You have already done more than we could ask. I have been watching you ever since you started looking after my daughter. You are the most compassionate doctor I have ever met. It is only that we have no family here in Mbala. The way she is, I doubt there is much to hope for. If I lost her from here, there will be no one to help me. It will be easier on the family if she went and died in my home in Kasama. Her husband is only a child. He is a poor fisherman on Lake Tanganyika. I wouldn't let my son in-law bare this burden here," He spoke plainly about the prognosis.

"The ambulance is going to Kasama to pick blood. They could give them a lift," the nurse on duty explained.

Dr Marximillian could no longer hold Rhoda on the ward. With a sad heart, he bade farewell to the first patient he met at ACH. She had been kept specifically for him; however, he couldn't help her. He was deeply disturbed for not being able to save Rhoda. He didn't understand why God had not answered his prayers concerning this patient. He wrote a letter to his colleagues at the central hospital explaining her condition and the treatment she needed. He still had hope Rhoda would live.

After seeing Rhoda off, Marx headed for the operating theatre. Three cases were waiting for him in theatre. These were; a caesarean section, intestinal obstruction in a two week old baby and Peritonitis in a Tanzanian woman.

Marx entered theatre still thinking about Rhoda. He met a cheerful nurse selling assorted spices to her colleagues in theatre. One spice drew Marx's attention.

"Is that Masala spice," he asked.

"It is Doctor. This is the best spice to use in beans. Get some for your home," she answered.

"This spice cures impotence and increases Libido tenfold. It is an aphrodisiac," he replied with a grin on his face.

Those that had already bought the spice were stopped in their tracks upon hearing Marx's comments. The men stood up to inspect this wonder spice curiously.

"Are you serious doctor," one nurse who had bought four bottles asked. "I don't want to wake things home that I won't handle."

"Let sleeping dogs lie," another commented.

"Why don't you try a small experiment with the guys in theatre?" Marx suggested. "Aphrodisiac comes from the Greek, aphrodisiakon pertaining to Aphrodite, the Greek goddess of love. You could also try Masala tea, it is an aphrodisiac too."

"I don't follow," she said.

"Yes, cook rice with chilemba and spicy it with an overdose of Masala and see what happens," a male nurse answered.

"Are sure, you will all eat just the rice. I don't want to be a witness in court," she laughed.

Marx hurried for the male change room. The team was still discussing the therapeutic dose of Masala spice when he finished the caesarean section. Everyone was *Marximused* to see him emerge out so soon.

The next operation took him till 2pm. The medical students had joined him for this operation. O'Neill and Ethel scrubbed in. The patient had crossed into Zambia from Tanzania. She lived in Mtula, a border town. The findings in the abdomen amazed Dr Marximillian's worn out mind. It was a miracle, she was alive.

She had suffered perforated peptic ulcers that Marx estimated to have been a week old. The abdomen was full of copious amount of foul smelling pus. Every segment of intestine was firmly adhered in the abdomen. There was no piece Marx could examine freely.

"How are you able to tell this was caused by perforated peptic ulcer disease?" O'Neill asked.

"By following the policeman of the abdomen," he answered looking at Ethel's *Marximesmerized* face.

"I didn't know ulcers could be this bad. Her abdomen had two litters of pus and she managed to walk from Mtula into Kawimbe and finally Mbala. She should thank God you were here. I can't believe my own eyes, she was rotting alive. We could have even found maggots in this abdomen," Ethel remarked in shock.

"Who is the police man of the abdomen?" the *Marximused* nurse asked.

"Dr O'Neil will tell us," said Dr Marximillian looking at his students.

"It is this material here," Ethel answered pointing at a thick fatty sheet like piece in the abdomen.

"It is the greater Omentum," O'Neil smiled.

"Omentum is Latin for apron. It is a large apron like fold that hangs down from the stomach, passing in front of the small intestines and reflects on itself to ascend to the transverse colon. It plays an important role in the immune system and it may also physically limit the spread of infection inside the abdomen. It can often be found wrapped around areas of infection or trauma, like in our case here. This is why it is sometimes referred to as simply the police man of the abdomen," Dr Marximillian explained holding the omentum in his hands.

He concluded the surgery after washing the abdomen thoroughly with saline and asked Ethel to write the operation notes. She had a beautiful handwriting that Marx liked.

"Why didn't we start with the baby," the theatre nurse asked.

"The father was not around to sign the consent," O'Neil answered. "Let me go and check whether he has come. He had not yet left Mpulungu when we came to theatre."

***

Dr Marximillian was only able to operate on the two week old baby at 8pm. He had stayed on in the hospital waiting for the child's father to arrive. He didn't have much to do in his room at Giza.

He was joined in theatre by his gorgeous students; Joan, Jessica and Selym. They walked into the operating room like models. Joan's blue scrubs incredibly defined her unblemished sexy female contours. She covered her head like an Arab girl. Only her cute eyes could be seen. Jessica and Selym too dressed to punish Marx's poor heart. He was glad, he had suffered occupational burnout.

The anaesthetist placed the miniature baby on the operating table. Its abdomen was grossly distended.

"My Gosh, it is so small, poor thing," Jessica remarked.

"Why can't disease choose its victims fairly?" bemoaned Joan.

"Life is just so cruel, just look at the way it is wriggling," remarked Selym.

"It wants its mother," said Joan.

"Girls, it is not a thing; she is a human being too. Please don't refer to her as 'IT'," the theatre nurse spoke up looking at the girls.

While the girls discussed babies, Dr Marximillian and Jessica stepped onto the operating table. Marx proceeded to map out his planed incision line. It was nearly 9pm by now. It was dark outside.

"This is a cruel operation doc. How do you feel cutting up a two week old baby?" Joan asked concerned.

"The first time I operated on a day old, I got sick on the Table. The operation was for intestinal obstruction. Thank God the baby lived. It is never a nice thing to do. However, when it is the only thing left to do in order to save a life, it must be done regardless how one feels about it," Marx replied looking at Joan.

The nurse passed the surgical knife to Dr Marximillian. He made an incision from the sternum down to the umbilicus. Within a few minutes clear fluid came gashing out from the abdomen accompanied by coils of tiny intestines.

Joan and Selym were dozing at the foot end of the operating table. They sat on chairs on either side of a small table used for writing theatre notes. Jessica looked at her sleepy friends. She was exhausted too. It had been a long day. Marx decided to operate without teaching. He was tired too. He didn't want to keep the baby under anesthesia for more than twenty minutes. As soon as he had mapped out the pathology inside the baby's abdomen, he concluded the operation and sent his girls to the hostels.

"Good night Dr Marximillian," Jessica called out as she left the female change room with a sleepy voice.

"Good night love," Marx answered. "Where are the others?"

"They have left me," she answered.

Marx completed his theatre notes and headed for the male change room. He bade farewell to his night theatre crew after he had changed.

"Good night doc. I hope they don't call you back at midnight for a ruptured uterus or sigmoid volvulus," the theatre nurse called out from the scrub room.

"I have reached a burnout my dear," he answered.

"You have been working 24/7 ever since you arrived. Have some rest," she advised.

Marx emerged into the wide corridor into which all the wards opened to, including theatre. He looked right towards surgical ward, children's ward at the far end of the western wing then to a spot he had resuscitated a woman with a ruptured uterus just the previous day. He decided to turn left and walk towards the car park to fetch the driver who would take him to his cold room at the Inn.

He turned right into another corridor just opposite the outpatient department. He pondered over the Architect's mind for choosing different ground elevations for the hospital in his design. The Outpatient building was built four meters below where he stood. Marx steadied his tired legs along the corridor's fifteen degree descent to the car park. It was dark and chilly outside. At the far end, the corridor made a sharp left turn and disappeared between the physiotherapy building on the right and the outpatient block on the left. Marx stopped momentarily like someone who had forgotten something. "I've not told the parents what we found. They must be very anxious," he murmured to himself.

With a matter like this weighing on his mind, Dr Marximillian knew he wouldn't be able to find sleep. He turned around and retraced his path and headed back for the surgical ward.

***

"I knew you would come back," said Isabelle when she saw him enter the ward. "I kept a snack for you and a Cola."

"What are you doing here? Aren't you supposed to be on your nights off?" Marx asked surprised to see the chief's daughter on duty. "Thank you for thinking about me. I am hungry, thirsty and tired; you are the only one who thinks about me in the whole world."

"You like that question. You asked me that when we first met. Now, what are you doing here? Hope not chasing the Mayor's daughter," she answered laughing.

"Jealousy ah," Marx remarked. "You've done well to be here, we need to explain to the parents what we found in the abdomen of the baby we just operated on.

Isabelle hurriedly found the parents and took them to the nurse's station. She gave them chairs and sat on a wide sofa next to Marx overlooking a wide window. They could see the baby on the acute bay from this wide glass window. Isabelle translated Dr Marximillian's every word with genuine compassion in her voice. The father nodded and shook his head from side to side as she talked. His wife sobbed silently by his side.

"We found a growth in the space between the liver and the right kidney. It had numerous abnormal blood vessels growing around it. It is a growth that resembles what we see in cases of cancers. However, I am not saying your child has a cancer. I have no evidence to suggest that. Just because a growth resembles a cancer does not make it a cancer. Therefore, we have collected a small piece of skin from the growth and will be sent to the pathologist in order to confirm what that mass was." Dr Marximillian spoke slowly allowing his beautiful translator to explain to the anxious parents.

"Do you think this baby will survive that water secreting tumor you described?" Isabelle asked when the couple had left them.

"You want a spiced answer or cold blooded truth?" Marx asked drawing her close to his chest.

"Mm, forget it. I am the next patient," she said after a moment's thought.

It was midnight by now. Marx was extremely exhausted.

"Yes, your text," he answered.

"Don't dose on me again," she giggled pulling his arm. "I brought my x-rays."

She stood up to fetch her x-rays. When she returned, she found Marx watching her Chishimba Falls photos.

"I was beautiful when I was young," she said sitting down.

"You are beautiful. You will always be beautiful," said Marx. Their eyes met. She looked down.

He knew if he sat long enough there, she would ask him a very difficult question; the *'Do you love me,'* rocket science question. She had a strong sense of déjà vu when she sat around him like that. He decided to stand and bade her goodnight. She resisted him from standing for a moment but soon allowed him. She told him she would go away for two weeks to Kitwe. She wanted him to promise he would still be around when she returned.

A Brush With The Mafia

It was a cold Friday morning in Mbala, the first day of April. Dr Marximillian showed no signs of slowing down. A major ward round was waiting for him at ACH. There were many patients anxiously looking forward to the doctor's round.

Dr Marximillian arrived in surgical ward in high spirits. His students were ready for him.

"This is Mr. Sinkamba. He is 81 years old; he was admitted last night for failure to pass urine. He is a known patient followed up for prostate enlargement for the past two years at this hospital," Jessica presented the first patient.

"What are the signs and symptoms of prostatic enlargement?" Dr Marximillian asked his students.

"Frequency; usually patients start going to the toilet more often than is usual for them," Kasonde answered.

"Hesitance; this is when urine delays to come out once the patient reaches the toilet," Kaluba answered.

"Poor stream; in patients with enlarged prostates, urine falls just near their feet. They can no longer shoot several meters away as they did when they were boys," Joan answered.

"Excellent; Are there any other symptoms you can remember?" Dr Marximillian asked.

"They also experience continuous dribbling of urine after they finish urinating," Felix answered.

"It is referred to as post micturition dribbling," said Joan smiling.

"Well done everyone. Jessica, follow up the laboratory result for Mr. Sinkamba. Tomorrow we will discuss management of prostate disease," Dr Marximillian told his students.

"I will sir," she answered.

"Mr. Sinkamba, I will see you when all the results are in. I would like to discuss the results with you and the treatment you will need," Dr Marximillian explained. "Who is this young man by your bed side?"

"Thank you doctor," Mr. Sinkamba answered. "This is my grandson. He is the one helping me. I am all by myself now. This disease has troubled me too much."

The old man lay on a bed at the back of the ward. His cloths smelt of urine. His seventeen year old grandson looked worried seeing his friend was ill. Among the Mambwe people, grandsons treated their grandfathers simply as best friends. This unique relationship existed across many cultures in Zambia.

The team walked away to see other patients on the ward that morning. It was a busy Friday. Everyone, including the students was planning for the weekend ahead. Marx thought about the old man as they walked away.

"It is a paradox how twisted life can be; when we are young we rely on others to take care of us. When we get old, we become young again, needing others to care for us," He explained

"I feel for that small boy, I am sure he does not even go to school," said Jessica.

"He probably lives alone with his grandfather. I am sure he cooks and even washes clothes for his grandfather. Village life is cruel," Joan bemoaned.

By now, the team had arrived in the female surgical ward. There was a patient that the relatives had declined surgery. She had been on the ward for a week and the condition continued to deteriorate. Dr Marximillian had diagnosed her with peritonitis and planned her for immediate surgery unfortunately her mother and the rest of the family declined surgery.

When Dr Marximillian approached her bed, he didn't like what he saw. The infection had spread into the patient's chest. The right lung was unable to allow in air. It had become like a wet sponge. The abdomen was grossly distended. Marx tapped on it and it resonated like a drum. The intestines had become blocked too. She had complicated into intestinal obstruction. A nazo- gastric tube from her nose drained copious amounts of dark green bile. She laboured with every breath she took. She was dying.

While Dr Marximillian was still on the ward, the patient's father arrived from Kasama. He had not seen his daughter since she was taken ill. He requested the nurses to allow him to see the doctors and find out for himself what he had heard on phone from his family about his daughter's illness.

"Doctor, I am the father to your patient with a swollen abdomen. I have just arrived from Kasama. Please explain to me what is wrong with my daughter," he asked.

Dr Marximillian decided to seize this opportunity to show the family what was going on inside the abdomen. He excused himself and told the man he needed to collect a sample to show him. When the family consented, Dr Marximillian asked the nurses and his students to place screens around the patient's bed and to give him a sixty millilitre syringe.

"Why do you want to do a speculum examination on the patient Dr Marximillian?" the nurse asked.

"Watch and learn," he answered.

He inserted a large bore needle in the space between the Uterus and the rectum through the vagina. A thick porridge like fluid filled the syringe. The students were *Marximesmerized.*

"This is called culdocentesis," he announced.

"Oh my god, It is pus; it smells awful; she would have been discharged by now had she accepted the operation when she came last week. I was here when Dr Kalunda admitted her and ordered laparotomy stat but the family refused," the nurse remarked closing her nose.

Marx walked to where the family sat on the benches next to the nurse's station. He asked Joan to hold a small dish and squeezed out the foul smelling pus for the relatives to see. They were terrified with what they saw and some looked away.

"Don't look away. You are the same people that refused the operation last week. This is what is killing your relative. Had the operation been done last week, she would have been discharged by now. You people never learn. Look at what your stubbornness has caused," the nurse rebuked the family.

"Sister," Dr Marximillian tried to intervene.

"I am very angry with this family doc. Forgive me. One week is too long. Look at the poor woman," she returned into the ward to clear the screens from the patient's bed.

"I am sorry sir, forgive the nurse. She was only expressing her concern for your daughter," Marx apologized for the nurse's reaction.

"She is right. We have interfered with your professional work," the father answered. "Like I said, I have just arrived; I didn't know her condition was this bad.

"Can you still operate on her in the condition she is," a medical student asked.

"I must say, we don't accept blood, however you can operate on her," the patient's father gave his position on blood transfusion.

Marx left the ward with his students after booking the patient for surgery. It was nearly lunch time by now. The Community Executive Officer, CEO, had asked to see Marx over lunch in his office.

*** ***

Marx walked from surgical ward and turned left into the wide corridor stretching in front of the wards on one side and the car park on the other. He passed several patients seated on benches waiting for their x-rays. It was cloudy outside and chilly. The exotic trees around the car park looked beautiful. Drivers were washing the advanced life support ambulance at the far end of the car park.

Marx turned left from the corridor towards the *CEO's* office. He wondered what she was calling him for. He entered the flamboyant office and found her lovely secretary, Idah, busy at her desk.

"Good afternoon Dr Marximillian," she greeted him.

"Good afternoon Idah," he answered. "Is she in?"

"Please go in, she is expecting you," she whispered.

Dr Marximillian tapped on the door and pushed on it. He found the CEO, seated behind a large executive table. She was flipping through a pile of papers on her desk.

"Ah, there he is…the man himself. Please make yourself comfortable. This is my office," she said when Marx entered the office.

"Thank you," Marx answered sitting down on a large sofa. "You have a beautiful office."

"How are you settling down in our community? I have heard about your exploits. Everyone is talking about you. We are very happy to have you," she said.

"I am flattered," he answered. "I have a very sick girl on the ward. Only a few minutes ago did the relatives consent for surgery."

"I heard about her in the morning report. Don't touch her if you feel she won't make it," she advised.

"I was thinking of doing a culdocentesis at 3pm. She has three litres pus in her abdomen. I would never forgive myself to sit back and do nothing while she deteriorates towards an untimely death," he answered.

"Exactly the reason why I called you," she started. "We worry so much about patients, yet no one worries anything about us doc."

"That is kind of true," he agreed vaguely.

"Doc, this is the time to make money. These patients will always be there. I know of a consultant who died in a guest house not too long ago. He was a very good doctor. He never wanted anything to do with administrative work. All he cared about were his patients and his ward work. He worked faithfully for twenty years. Then one day, he fell ill and he couldn't work anymore. Over the years, new people who didn't know our poor friend were employed and posted to his hospital in human resource. Then these morons removed the poor consultant of surgery from the payroll. He had no money to pay rent. He had not yet built himself a house. Like every good doctor, he was too busy caring for his patients and forgot about himself. As things turned out, his landlord evicted him and he was thrown onto the streets," she explained visibly angry.

"That is scary doc," Marx remarked thinking about his own troubles.

"This story makes me angry each time I share it with fellow doctors. We work hard. We spend forty years of our lives studying. Yet these fools in the hospital think we are the same. That is why personally, I don't have any kind words for morons who think we are the same," she rattled on. "Look at me. I am over forty now and without a child of my own. I was too busy with school and forgot about a visit to the labour ward. I am too old to conceive now."

"But you don't look forty at all. I would say late twenties or thirty one to be more precise," said Marx sitting upright in his sofa.

"I am flattered," she said and let out a bright smile. "I am old Dr Marximillian."

"What happened to our colleague?" Marx asked returning to the subject.

"He died like a vagabond," she stated. "An ordinary local fellow, an Inn Keeper, took pity on him and gave him two rooms at the Inn. He died shortly after that. Every time I think about this, his death pains me like he was my own brother."

"That is a very sad story," said Marx.

"It is all about the money doc. None of these assholes gives a fuck what happens to us. We are always here closed behind these cruel walls we call the hospital and work our asses out 24/7. We deceive ourselves and call it dedication to work. It is a lie. The Oncall allowance you receive just pays for five days in a month at a rate of One dollar an hour. That means you give twenty five days in a month for free. No one pays you for those extra days. Each doctor ought to be Oncall one day a week plus a weekend call. Unfortunately there are so many doctors being paid call allowances for calls they do not do. We burn our asses for free and we deceive ourselves by calling it dedication to our patients. We are woken up at night to save someone dying while these scumbags sleep. Take this hospital for instance, do you know how many cadres work here?" she asked flipping through a large pile of files on her desk.

"How many general workers does the hospital employ?" Marx asked.

"Four hundred and yet there are only four doctors. Four f**kn doctors to care for a population of twenty four thousand people; the core business of this institution. Yet there are four hundred to mop floors, empty bins, cut seasonal grass, fix doors and repair non functioning hospital equipment. It is no wonder hospitals are so unmanageable," she spoke with a bitter tone in her voice revealing lines of advancing age around her eyes and lips.

"It is the reason the Army demands compulsory military training for everyone planning on joining them. The army can't stand the indiscipline of civilians," said Marx. "I see what you have to put up with."

"They are a pain in the ass. We bring people to life while they sit around all day. We give people second chances to walk this earth. We are not like those morons who would send someone to jail for stealing just a little meal to nourish his starving tummy," she spoke with obvious sarcasm in her voice. "Honestly, how many people are needed to clean these floors? You just need two to drive those motorized vacuum cleaners and outsource a maintenance company to deal with the rest. Have you seen those little cars they use to clean large airport floors? That is what we need."

"I have," said Marx wondering where this chat was leading to.

"I strongly think developers of artificial intelligence should keenly exploit this area," she suggested. "Imagine robots cleaning your hospital floors and handling medical waste. Their efficiency could be enhanced by fitting hospitals with smart floors. We wouldn't need to dig out entire floors; we just need the technology incorporated in tiling materials."

"What a ratio, one doctor to six thousand people; we are an endangered species," remarked Marx still thinking about the doctor to patient ratio in the Abercorn population. "It's not only the sick who need a doctor you know."

"It is time to quit, a time to leave the sickening wards and head out to make money. Get plots and build; spend whole days at your plot. Leave the sick to care for themselves. Or join a crazy programme with a fancy name and move to head office to coordinate it. If you are into maize, shift to Mkushi and build storage facilities and stock up on maize. Treating malaria and diarrhea will not help us. Let us apply our brains at the bigger picture. Look at Dr Ben Carson; he has finally seen the bigger picture. He quit his practice as professor of neural surgery. He now wants to be president of America. Though I think he will lose to Donald Trump. The guy inspired many of us to become doctors. Did you read his books; Gifted Hands and Think Big? The world doesn't need doctors. If you want to work, make sure you don't give out your hard earned skills for free," Dr Lillian Lupiya- Mikhailov continued to corrupt Marx's compassionate mind.

"Lately, I have been questioning myself along those lines," Marx admitted but would not share his debt and other social mayhem he was going through.

"I own and have built houses in every provincial capital in this country. I have sixty two flats in total and a big farm in Mkushi. These properties are more valuable to me than a PhD. I laugh when I meet friends going to study for PhDs in some disgusting little known disease. PhDs are for your grand Children. You need to level the playing field for them. Give your children leverage, the education you have attained is enough for you. Build Apartments doc at doctor's standard. Don't waste time chasing a PhD in surgery. Leave that for your great grand children; PhDs will be their toys to play with. Children cannot inherit your PhD," she let out a sardonic grin and laughed.

"Sixty two, how did you do that?" Marx asked thoughtfully.

"They are proceeds from my three failed foreign marriages," she said looking down. "My last husband was a Russian Mafia. We met in

Moscow. He wanted me to invest part of his money in Africa. He was brutally murdered in our hotel room. I narrowly escaped."

She broke down behind her desk and choked on her saliva. She reached out for the fridge in the office and poured two glasses of Vodka. She passed one to Marx and smiled.

"A cola for me please," he said.

"Ah, theatre man; It is nearly half past three. Don't forget your dying patient in surgical ward," she said putting down her empty glass of Vodka. "I am now forty one. I have houses but no child to show for it. It pains me when I think about it. If you need flats to buy, come and see me. You are welcome any time."

***

Marx left the office and walked towards the operating theatre. He was not sure whether he agreed with Dr Lillian Lupiya-Mikhailov's ideology. Marx had a weakness for people. He felt sorry for the workers she had trashed. Marx respected people regardless their job description. He always

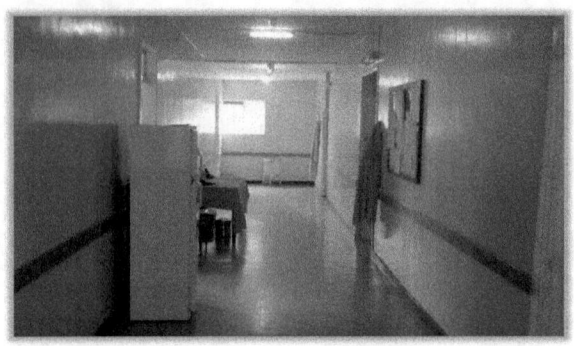

thought of himself as a human first and as a doctor second. He was convinced all people were equal. Their various job descriptions and qualifications were merely tools to do a job. However, he found Dr Lillian Lupiya-Mikhailov's ideology irresistible owing to his recent woes. She corrupted his mind irreversibly and he was afraid, he would lose his temperament. The writing on the wall was indelible.

He wasn't a saint, and knew he couldn't hope for a reward in heaven. He would ensure he had his reward delivered on earth. He was convinced it was all about the money like Mikhailov had put it. He thought about her name for a while and murmured to himself, "Lillian is derived from the Flower name Lily; symbol of innocence, purity and beauty. This Vodka girl is the exact opposite of her name. She is now a Mafia, poor girl."

He pushed the wide double door leading into theatre. It swung open and ushered him in, the students were already in theatre waiting for him. He turned right immediately into the foot wear change room and traded his shoes for the operating room Clogs. Then he walked towards the change room at the far end of the corridor. He found the anaesthetist waiting for him in the change room.

"Doctor Marximillian, why are you bringing this dying patient to theatre? I don't think this patient can survive anesthesia let alone the surgery," the anaesthetist stated when they met in the change room. "Why can't you just leave her alone? Everyone can see that she is dying."

"I am not planning on opening her abdomen. Nonetheless, her family has already consented to what I intend to do. They are aware about death as a possible outcome. However, if you are uncomfortable, I will send for the other anaesthetist," Marx answered and walked away to join his students.

Jessica sat on a chair beside a wide work table. Marx walked in and sat opposite her. Joan sat on a bench just to the left of the entrance into the duty room. She rested her head in her palms. She looked beautiful as always in her blue scrubs. Felix sat with her. Johnny and George stood and leaned against an old wooden cupboard on the far right corner. It was 4pm by now.

"How did you convince the anaesthetist into accepting this sick patient? You know he is difficult that one," the theatre nurse asked when she entered the duty room.

"I told him to leave if he felt uncomfortable," Marx answered.

"How are we going to know what is causing the pus if we don't open her abdomen?" Jessica asked.

"That is a good question. We won't know the cause. She wouldn't survive a laparotomy. I hope this would help stabilize her for definitive surgery later," Dr Marximillian explained admiring Jessica. He loved these girls, only they didn't know.

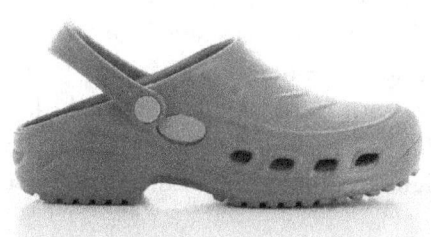

"Please explain the procedure to us," Joan asked sitting upright. Her virgin breasts stood elegantly on her chest. They were kept in check by a sexy white brassiere.

Marx looked at her chest and could see her inner aspects through the V shaped collar in her scrub. She caught his prowling eye and slowly adjusted her top with a gentle smile. Marx felt a tremor run up his spine. It reminded him his mortal nature. He felt vulnerable in the event anyone of these beautiful girls chose to seduce him. He knew he couldn't refuse.

"The procedure will be exactly similar to what we did on the ward except, it will be on a large scale. We will make an opening into the abdomen via the vagina. We will enter behind or posterior to the cervix into a space found between the uterus and the rectum. This space is referred to as the recto-uterine pouch or simply, pouch of Douglas. It is the lowest point in the body when a woman lies down," he explained looking at Joan. Their eyes met and she looked down.

She had beautiful white eyes and lovely black eyebrows against a smooth baby face without blemishes. Marx thought she would have looked prettier had she chosen a career in law or Banking.

"The patient is ready," the nurse came to announce.

"Joan and Jessica, you will scrub in with me," Marx chose his faithful surgeons.

"No, it is our turn today. Joan and Jessica always assist you," Johnny protested.

"You are right," Marx answered him. "And that is why I don't change the winning team. This is not some kind of changing turns game. I have been building a team ever since I arrived here. The girls have always been with me and assisted me in many complicated cases. They have not dodged theatre like many of you boys. They have shown great eagerness to learn. I need to use the skills I have taught them in this operation. I don't want to start teaching someone raw. The patient is very sick," Marx defended his girls with a firm voice.

They were very delighted to learn how he felt about them.

"Thank you doc for shutting the guys off, they always think dirty things about us. They think we come to theatre to see you for other things," said Joan laughing at Johnny.

"I know. Have you ever seen the homunculus of a man?" Marx asked.

"No," Joan answered.

"A naked woman sits on it," Marx answered with a grin.

They all burst out laughing. They emerged into the operating room after crossing the scrubbing area.

***

The patient lay on the table barely breathing. A black oxygen mask covered her mouth and nose. The anaesthetist stood by the head end angry. Marx walked in with his students talking cheerfully.

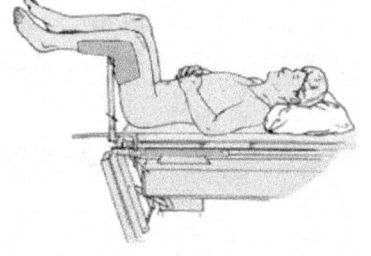

It was quiet outside. The visiting hour was over and people were hurrying, returning to their various homes in family groups. The sun flew low on the western horizon. A cold breeze swept across the hospital. Dusk was upon the small town of Mbala. Some discussed this patient as they walked back to their homes. It was clear even to lay people, the patient was dying. The anesthetist was angry because Marx had brought a hopeless case to theatre.

The nurse positioned her instruments table on the right side of Dr Marximillian. He sat on a stool at the foot end of the patient. Joan stood closely to his left. Her waist rubbed against Marx's left shoulder. They stood between the patient's legs which were placed on special supports and strapped at the knees.

"This is called the lithotomy position," Marx explained.

"Like they do in labour ward," Joan remarked.

"That is correct Dr Joan," Marx agreed looking up at Joan. She was a tall girl and towered gracefully above his head. "Lithotomy is a medical term referring to a common position for surgical procedures and medical examinations involving the pelvis and lower abdomen, as well as a common position for childbirth like Joan said. The lithotomy position involves the positioning of an individual's feet above or at the same level as the hips, often in stirrups, with the perineum positioned at the edge of the examination table or operating table as in our case here."

"It is a very bad position when it is done with a fully conscious person," Jessica remarked. She was scrubbed in and stood on the patient's right waiting for instructions from Dr Marximillian.

"You are right. Actually patients have reported feeling a loss of control and increased sense of vulnerability when examined in the lithotomy position because they cannot see the area being examined. Other, equally effective positions have been suggested for examinations of conscious patients," Dr Marximillian explained.

"That is better, I would cry on you if you placed me in this position Dr Marx," said Joan laughing.

"I am sure he wouldn't want to do it under such conditions too," the anaesthetist remarked joining the conversation.

"Sir, she is only a child," the theatre nurse came to Joan's rescue. Everyone burst out laughing.

"It is good to have you back sir. I am sorry about our little fight earlier. You know I enjoy working with you," said Marx looking across at the anaesthetist.

"You are welcome doc. I was wrong," he answered.

"Now back to Dr Joan's position," he paused for a reaction from his beautiful assistants.

"No doc, I fear this position. You can kill someone," she remarked laughing.

"Don't worry, our patient won't die," he answered with a grin on his face. "References to this position have been found in some of the oldest known medical documents including versions of the Hippocratic Oath. The position is named after the ancient surgical procedure for removing Kidney stones and bladder stones via this route, the perineum. The position is perhaps most recognizable as the 'often used' position for childbirth: the patient is laid on the back with knees bent, positioned above the hips, and spread apart through the use of stirrups. The position is frequently used and has many obvious benefits from the doctor's perspective."

He paused to allow for a reaction from his team.

"Doc, it also has many domestic benefits," the anaesthetist remarked.

"Dr Joan and Dr Jessica are not yet 19. You will confuse them," Marx warned the anaesthetist and rose from his stool.

"That is not true sir. We are big girls. We'll turn 23 next month," Jessica protested.

"Then I will continue with my lecture; 'benefits of the Lithotomy position', uncensored," he smiled. "Most notably the position provides good visual and physical access to the Perineal region and most important, to the vagina. The position is used for procedures ranging from simple pelvic exams, like we did on the ward, to complex surgeries like the one we are performing right now. However, new observations and scientific findings, combined with a greater sensitivity to patient needs have raised awareness of the physical and psychological risks the position may pose for prolonged surgical procedures, pelvic examinations, and, most notably, childbirth. A Cochrane Review found that the lithotomy position may not be the ideal position for child birth, noting that while it makes care easier for midwives and doctors by placing the patient in an easily accessible position, it is often harder on birthing mothers as use of the lithotomy position can narrow the birth canal by up to a third. In lieu of the lithotomy position, the Cochrane Review recommended birthing mothers make informed choices about birthing positions and find the position that is most comfortable for them."

"It is the same in the home, there are now many positions to choose from," the anaesthetist continued with his domestic discourse. "Actually doc, these young girls nowadays, know sophisticated positions that would make your eyes fill up with a torrent of tears and easily kill you from a heart attack."

The theatre nurse burst out laughing. The boys joined in laughing on top of their voices.

"Leave my doctors alone. These are angels. They do not know of any positions you are talking about," Marx defended his lovely assistants with a firm voice. However a grin on his face gave him away.

By now, the runner had brought twenty litters of saline and another twenty litters of distilled water from the laboratory. Dr Marx opened the posterior fornix and introduced two large drainage tubes. Copious amounts of foul smelling pus came gushing out.

Felix turned on the suction machine and filled three litres of brownish white pus within ten minutes. Marx passed one drainage tube to Jessica and instructed her to pour saline through the tube at will. George, who had been very quiet all this while, assisted Jessica on the right side. Marx passed the second tube to Kaoma and her assistant, Kaluba. Joan assisted Marx at the perineum and with positioning of the tubes into the vagina.

"Poor woman, she is rotten inside. If she survives, she should thank God you came. We would not have touched her if it weren't for you. You are a brave man doc, you really are," said the anaesthetist looking at Marx who was busy working between the patient's legs.

"You see why I needed all of you here. Where are the others, the priest and Shifu? Were they not with you in the duty room?" Marx asked.

"They went back to the hostels. They thought you only wanted Joan and Jessica," Kaluba answered.

"That is the reason I do not teach surgery to lazy students. These are dangerous skills to place in the hands of malingerers." He stood up and let Joan continue guiding the abdominal irrigation.

After several litters of saline, the job was finally done. The patient's abdomen flattened out and her breathing showed some remarkable improvements. Marx was pleased with the work his team had done.

He had completely forgotten about Dr Lillian Lupiya- Mikhailov's dissertation but now her words had returned to harangue him. He had just saved a life, however he would earn zero dollars for the work he had just done. And since he was not a saint, he would neither receive a reward here on earth nor in heaven. He was almost convinced his work was a total waste of his valuable time.

He left the hospital at 10pm pondering over Dr Lillian Lupiya-Mikhailov's words. He found the restaurant closed at the Inn. There was no food. He was hungry and tired. He was too busy saving lives to think about his supper. He found a pack of biscuits in his traveler's bag and made himself some coffee.

"What if she was right?" he thought, sipping his black coffee.

After finishing his coffee, he lay on the bed and reflected on the conversation he had with Dr Lillian Lupiya- Mikhailov. He didn't agree with her call to doctors to leave the wards. The real problem he saw was failure by *The System* to attract a few good doctors to the ward. Patients needed good doctors. He pondered over the reasons that made even a few good doctors to leave the ward. He concluded it was all about the money. Vulture doctors were always well fed while a few good doctors starved. The former scavenged carcasses in high places where they gathered and gorged themselves on succulent marinated flank steak with impunity.

Marx belonged to a school of thought which considered Medicine to be a science practiced transparently on the hospital ward or the doctor's office. Unfortunately, money was kept far away from the ward, thereby forcing even a few good doctors out of the ward. It was all about the money.

Marx's colleagues had repeatedly argued never to support the common practice by public hospitals to meddle into private practice. Insisting that patients who sort private practice wanted individualized care and control over who would attend them. They went further to argue that, anyone who paid money for his health care ought to be given the freedom to choose his or her doctor from a menu of a few good doctors;

After wrestling with these thoughts for a while, Dr Marximillian decided to document his views on a voice recorder.

"In hospitals where Scavengers and Vultures were on the menu, a detailed warning, in form of credentials, ought to be made available to patients to help them make informed choices," he spoke into his phone's mouth piece. It was quiet outside except for numerous frogs that were croaking all around Giza. "It is Foolish to pay money for private practice or High Cost Care and not know who would operate on your child or perform a Caesarean section on your wife. No hospital has ever operated on a patient; it is only doctors that operate on patients. Once people begin to have Choices on how they spent their hard earned health care money; on which doctor they entrusted their life to; a few good doctors would return to the wards in large numbers. No one walks into a restaurant only to have food forced on them. It is the freedom of choice from the menu that keeps the flow to the hungry man's clinic. At public institutions, the roster decides which doctor sees the patient. A public institution that makes people pay for the so called High cost services, must morally offer the best Doctor Menu money can buy to their patients. It would then be the duty of the Medical Aid provider to ensure lucrative incentives are kept on the ward to attract the best specialists to care for patients seeking individualized care. When this happens, all doctor's roads will lead back to the ward. No doctor will choose to remain dormant in a stupid office when the party was on the ward. Finest doctors, young and old, including vultures of course, would dust up their old white tuxedos and head back for the dance floor inside the ward. Good health care is all about the money. It is no wonder Britain and America pay colossal salaries to finest doctors poached from around the world. They need them on the ward to fuel the finest health care system money can buy."

In a Socialist Medicare System the state owns and operates health care facilities and employs the health care professionals, thus also paying for all health care services. In the United States, a national health system for Americans goes all the way back to the days of President Teddy Roosevelt, whose platform included health insurance when he ran for president in 1912. However, the idea for a national health plan didn't gain steam until it was pushed by U.S. President Harry S. Truman. On November 19, 1945, seven months into his presidency, Truman sent a message to Congress, calling for creation of a national health insurance fund open to all Americans. The plan Truman envisioned would provide health coverage to individuals, paying for such typical expenses as doctor visits, hospital visits, laboratory services, dental care and nursing services. Although Truman fought to get a bill passed during his term, he was unsuccessful and it was another twenty years before Medicare would become a reality.

President John F. Kennedy made his own unsuccessful push for a national health care program for seniors after a national study showed that 56% of Americans over the age of 65 were not covered by health insurance. But it wasn't until 1965, after legislation was signed by Lyndon B Johnson, that Americans started receiving Medicare health coverage. To date, Medicare continues to provide healthcare for those in need. By the end of 2014, there were approximately fifty million people receiving health coverage through a Medicare program in America. Benefits paid in 2013 amounted to 14% of the federal budget.

The matters Marx was wrestling with left his mind extremely exhausted. He fell asleep after a grueling mental review of the American Medicare and more recently, ObamaCare which offers Americans more benefits, rights and protection. It is officially referred to as the Patient Protection and Affordable Care Act or simply, the Affordable Care Act, ACA. This is a US healthcare reform law that expands and improves access to care and curbs spending through regulations and taxes. The ACA's main focus is on providing more Americans with access to affordable health insurance, improving the quality of healthcare and health insurance, regulating the health insurance industry, and reducing reckless health care spending in the US.

Highly skilled doctors are indispensable in the pursuit of provision of Quality Health Care. There can be no Quality Health Care without a system that attracts a few good doctors back to the wards to care for the sick. Creation of an affordable yet lucrative health care industry should take leave from prosperous football leagues in the world. Highly Skilled Professional players on the pitch attract funs and advertisers of the beautiful game, teams win the games. In football, money is placed on the pitch to attract the best players in the world. In Marx's world, Money was placed far from the ward, rendering most hospitals death traps. Even a few good doctors who had sacrificed all to care, where now being cruelly maligned and prevented from practicing their trade on the ward and save lives.

Fait Accompli

The next day, Saturday 2nd April, Marx got up early and watched his life burnout like a candle before him. Whereas for most people the week had come to an end, his had just started.

All his mates had turned out to be fair weather friends. He was all alone and broke. His Mbala vacation was beginning to wear him down. He considered calling off his medical tour and return to Lusaka. He knew each day that passed, he would acquire many more new patients and make it difficult for him to leave.

The hospital driver remembered to pick him that morning. He arrived in an old pick up that audibly begged to be taken to the garage. It was long overdue on its service. The car rocked the entire way to the hospital.

The sky was clear above. The road was slippery. The pot holes and ditches had been turned into water ponds. It rained cats and dogs the previous night. Marx admired the green grass by the road side. The fertile brown soils of Mbala supported amazing green vegetation all around the town.

After a tormenting drive, dodging pot holes in the gravel road to the hospital, the pickup came to a stop in the hospital car park, just in front of the surgical ward. Dr Marximillian rushed to see his post culdocentesis patient. He found her alive alright but only just; she looked gravely ill.

Just then, Joan and Jessica walked in. They looked enthusiastic as always.

"Our patient doesn't look well," he said.

"At least the distension is gone," said Jessica.

"Come, help me change her beddings. She is soiled," he said.

"Why don't we ask the nurses to do it?" Joan asked.

"I don't think they care. They could have changed this patient before we came," said Jessica.

They changed the beddings while the nurses watched from their duty room. They couldn't even walk in to stop a senior officer from doing their job. Marx left the girls to finish the notes while he attended a patient who had come to see him.

"Excuse me girls, let me see that man over there," Dr Marximillian said taking off his gloves.

The girls remained alone for a short while and filled the time with some chitchat.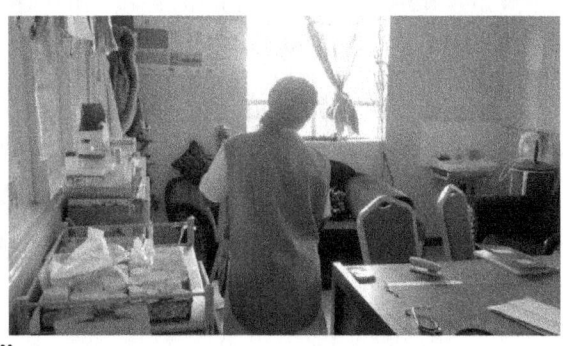

"Nursing has really gone to the dogs," Joan remarked. "Look at them; they are seated while Dr Marximillian does their work."

"These nurses are rude. They have no morals. It is no wonder they get assaulted on the wards," Jessica agreed with Joan.

"I used to admire nurses a lot when I was little. I had wanted to become a nurse and dress in that beautiful white uniform some day," said Joan.

"What happened?" Jessica asked.

"My uncle discouraged me, yet he was married to a nurse," Joan explained with a flush of nostalgia. "He used to call nurses well trained maids."

"That wasn't fair. My mom is a nurse. There are some nurses who are very good out there," said Jessica.

"I know; my uncle was just a crazy man. He was a mechanical engineer by profession. My uncle only regarded Engineers, Medical Doctors, Nuclear Physicists, Military Commanders and Generals to be the most educated people on earth. He hated Lawyers and called them well trained thieves."

When they had finished, Marx left with the girls. They walked chatting about nursing care among other things. In the corridor to gynecology ward, they were met by a woman carrying an ultrasound report. Many patients had by now known Dr Marximillian and could easily walk up to him for a consultation. The lady came over and gave Marx her report. He didn't like what he read.

"This lady has a ruptured ectopic pregnancy according to this ultrasound report," Marx remarked turning to his girls.

"How can it be ruptured when she looks stable like this?" Jessica asked. "Can a person walk and have a ruptured ectopic?"

"We learnt in class that ruptured ectopic cause acute abdomen," said Joan. "We were told patients come in shock and are critically ill. Surely this is a wrong diagnosis."

"You will learn something new today," said Marx smiling. "Books are written to offer guidance only."

"Can we do culdocentesis," Joan asked smiling.

"Excellent Dr Joan," Marx remarked leading the way.

They arrived in gynecology ward. The girls led the patient to the examination couch.

"We'll place her in Lithotomy position," she giggled.

"Explain to her. Do you remember what I said in theatre yesterday?" he asked

"It makes patients feel vulnerable because they cannot see the area being examined," Jessica explained.

"Excellent Dr Jessica," said Marx. "We don't want to scare our patient.

Patricia had travelled from Nsokolo village along Nakonde road, more than sixty kilometres from Abercorn Community Hospital on public transport. She had complained of abdomen pain for two weeks before presenting at ACH. At her local clinic, she was told she had ulcers and was given anti ulcers drugs. However, the symptoms worsened. She started experiencing episodes of black outs and when the clinic got tired of her, they told her to go to the hospital to scan her ulcers.

In the examination room, Marx sat on a stool with the patient placed in lithotomy position. He had difficult to perform the culdocentesis as the patient was uncooperative despite the girl's reassurances that everything would be alright. She kept closing her legs and moving backwards.

"Maybe that speculum is too big for her doc," Joan suggested looking at Marx.

"I see, you want a fight with me Dr Joan," Marx answered smiling at the girls. "It is the right size. Have you ever catheterized a grown man with an erect penis?"

"Doc, what are you implying?" Joan asked hiding behind Jessica.

"They are the same size," the midwife who had come to help answered.

"Hell no, that thing is cold and is made out of metal," Jessica protested.

"Thank you sister, these girls think I am cruel," said Marx rising from his chair. He smiled at the girls as he handed the speculum to the midwife. "Here, insert the speculum for me. This one is not cold."

The midwife gave the patient a firm lecture in her mother tongue on the synonyms of penises and speculums. She then drove the speculum without a groan from the patient. The girls thought she was cruel. They despised her methods and disagreed strongly with her speculum analogy. While the girls protested, Marx took his seat and inserted a large bore needle into Douglas' pouch and aspirated ten millilitres of dark blood.

"She has ruptured," Joan exclaimed.

"She is bleeding," said Jessica. "It is a DEFCON 2."

"Sister, inform theatre," said Marx standing up.

Soon after confirming the diagnosis, the team switched into emergency mode. Marx decided to pass through the radiology department to congratulate the sonographer who had written the report about the ruptured ectopic pregnancy. He arrived within a few minutes after a right turn from the wide corridor overlooking the car park.

"Who is Bruce?" he asked when he got into the department.

"I am here doc," he answered. "Is anything the matter?"

"I came to congratulate you on your incredible work. You have just saved a life," said Marx beaming with genuine excitement.

"What have I done doc?" Bruce asked confused.

"The woman you sent to me with a ruptured ectopic," he answered.

"I saw fluid in the pouch of Douglas and an ovarian mass. I concluded it must be an Ectopic." I am happy if you think so too," he answered.

"I do not think so; I know so… right now, I am on my way to the OR to operate on her. You are welcome to witness the operation," he explained. "Excellent work my friend, Keep it up."

Marx left Bruce *Marximesmerized*. No doctor had ever congratulated him for the work he did. This was a new experience. Marx had just brightened his dull Saturday morning. On the way to theatre, Jessica and Joan rushed to the hostels to fetch their scrubs and inform their mates on the operation scheduled for the OR. They were excited to have witnessed application of culdocentesis in diagnosing a ruptured ectopic pregnancy.

***

Marx spent his Saturday afternoon visiting little Poland. He was happy the operation for ectopic pregnancy had gone well.

After leavening the hospital, he walked into town to look for a restaurant open on Saturday. As was the custom in Mbala, the Sabbath brought business to a stand still for many. Marx's restaurant at the Inn was closed.

He searched for an eating place behind Ten Kwacha shopping complex. At Ten kwacha, he found the restaurant had run out of food. A cheerful lady at the counter directed Marx to a building not far from Ten Kwacha located along the hospital road, not far from the magnificent Catholic Church building in town. The architectural design was testimony of enduring building legacy of the Romans. It was undoubtedly the best master piece in Mbala. Marx was too hungry to inspect it closely. He reserved his curiosity for another day when he would visit in the company of his catholic students, Johnny the Priest and Sister Francis.

After a few turns, Marx found the restaurant. It was empty except for three young girls at the counter. Like most teen agers, they were busy playing on their cells phones and would not greet him. He quickly took charge of the atmosphere and lectured the poor girls on basic hospitality to strangers. He then ordered Nshima with fish.

One of the girls quickly disappeared through a dark passage at the back of the restaurant with his order. The walls were stained with ugly patches left behind by human hands. He wondered how the hands preparing his food looked like as he took a sit on an untidy table at the back. When his eyes had adjusted to focus more clearly in the dim light of the restaurant, he suddenly found himself surrounded by food debris, particles of hair and giant flies feasting on fish bones on a table not far from where he sat. When the waiter emerged from the dark passage with his meal, Marx fled the restaurant before she could get close to his table.

***

As was his habit, he awoke early the next morning and strolled into town towards the war memorial round about. He took a right turn and walked up hill towards little Poland, a beautiful residential area in Mbala. Soon after leaving the roundabout, he was met by a long motorcade. All the vehicles had their lights on. Marx's quick mind figured this to be a funeral procession. He stood to pay his last respects to the deceased he did not know. He knew it couldn't be any of his patients. God had been most gracious to him; he had not lost a patient since coming to Mbala.

'The deceased must have been a good person,' he thought, for there were many vehicles stretching endless as far as the eye could see. There were trucks and buses loaded with mourners. Several private cars joined the procession too. While he was thinking, a white car passed him and a rear tinted window opened. A voice called his name; he turned and saw a small pretty hand waving at him. "Isabelle," he called recognizing her hand.

The funeral convoy stretched on. The whole Mbala had turned up to pay their last respects. Marx couldn't wait any longer. He crossed the road and decided to take a taxi to the hospital. This funeral reminded him of his patients on the ward. On the way to the hospital, the taxi driver explained to Marx the mystery behind Ten Kwacha shopping complex. This driver was a cheerful man and made an excellent tour guide. Dr Marximillian would use his taxi for the remaining days of his stay in Mbala.

"Legend has it," he started explaining when they passed Ten Kwacha building. "This old man, the owner, started his business with only Ten Kwacha."

"Did he spend ten kwacha to build or Ten Kwacha was his total capital?" Marx asked.

"His total capital was Ten Kwacha, Ba sir," he explained. "He named his building Ten Kwacha to remind him how he started. That was a very long time ago. I wasn't even born. His story is an inspiration to many young people in Mbala."

"Incredible," Marx remarked. "That is equivalent to One Dollar. The size of a seed does not determine the height of the tree."

"That's right Ba sir," the taxi driver agreed. "I started my taxi business working for someone. Now I have five of my own and I have drivers who work for me. However, I still drive a taxi myself. I consider myself the sixth driver in my small fleet and my employees as work mates."

"You are an incredible man," Marx could not hide his admiration for this young entrepreneur. "I am a doctor at the Hospital."

"My aunt was admitted last night, is it possible you could help me see her," he asked upon learning his passenger was a doctor.

Dr Marximillian and his entrepreneur Taxi driver arrived at the hospital and went straight to see the patient. The hospital looked deserted when they arrived. It was Sunday and most departments were closed.

Marx led his driver to the high cost side ward were his aunt was admitted for diabetes. He then proceeded to see his post op patients on the ward.

He found his students, George and Shifu, on the ward inserting IV Cannulars on a new admission. They were dressed in military regalia. Dr Marximillian was not pleased with them.

"When you come on the wards, come in scrubs so that you can be identified properly. I keep my clinical coat here and I use it whenever I enter the wards," he advised the students.

"Our coats are in the nurse's duty room," Shifu answered.

"Then go and get them. You look like criminals," he told them.

He then turned to see the post Ectopic patient in the acute bay. She was out of danger. He told her he would discharge her the following day. She was delighted and thanked him for saving her life. In the corner, seated by the window, he reviewed the patient he had done auto transfusion. This was the patient he had resuscitated with his incredible team in the corridor by the car park. She was smiling when he stopped to shake her hand. She sobbed when he took her hand.

"You are fine now. God loves you my dear," he told her.

"Thank you for saving my life doctor," she said wiping her eyes. "When can I go home?"

"You are discharged," he told her. "However, you can go tomorrow so that you collect some medicine. Pharmacy is closed today."

He left soon after that and headed for the female surgical ward to see the culdocentesis patient from whom he had removed three litters of pus and the lady who had travelled from Chipapa in Tanzania to see him with perforated peptic ulcer disease.

The female surgical ward was located in the same building as the children's ward. The nurse on duty was a wonderful young lady. She stood immediately she saw Dr Marximillian and greeted him in the most respectful manner.

"Where did you do your training my dear?" he asked. "You are the first nurse who is properly trained I have met ever since I came here."

"Thank you sir," she answered. "I think charity begins at home."

"Are you implying, I shouldn't blame nursing school for rogue square pegs they are sending to hospitals nowadays," he asked fascinated with the adorable young nurse standing before him.

"I think the homes they come from are the ones tarnishing the image of many nursing schools," she answered.

"I have met very bad nurses in my life dear. Some so bad that you would think they came out of demon holes," he said. "I will make you nurse of the year when I have power to do so one day."

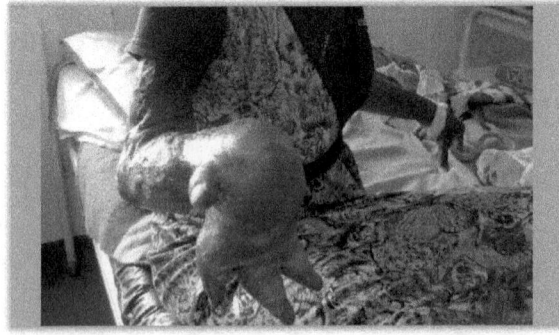

She smiled courteously at him and led the way into the ward pushing her trolley. She wore a bright white uniform and protected it with a neatly secured blue apron. Her white eyes surrounded by long dark eye lashes shone brightly with innocence. She was of median height and slim. Her feminine waist angled benevolently at the hip. Marx thought she was the most beautiful nurse he had ever set his eyes on.

The culdocentesis patient was still looking ill. However, she was beginning to sit with little support in bed. Next to her, the Tanzanian patient had fully recovered and couldn't wait to be told she could return to her home in Chipapa. Her mother, who had sat by her bed side since the day they arrived in Zambia, was delighted when Dr Marximillian discharged her daughter.

The next patient, Chola, sat on the edge of the bed breast feeding her lovely baby. Dr Marximillian had admitted her via casualty the previous day.

"How can we best help Chola Dr Marximillian? Should we just continue with wet saline soaks?" Marx's beautiful nurse asked.

"Rachael is this the way you pronounce your name?" he asked.

"Its Rachel," she answered. "You can call me Rachael, I don't mind."

"The best we can do for Chola in this hospital is to amputate her limb. However her mother and herself declined amputation when I saw her in casualty yesterday," Dr Marx explained.

"She has agreed to amputation. I read your admission notes. I talked with the family. They agreed to have the amputation," Rachel explained.

"Really, that is very good. Let's book her for tomorrow," said Marx excitedly. "Not only are you beautiful, you are a good counselor too."

"Thank you sir," she answered naively. "I am pleased you think so about me."

"I have a terrible toothache. It is giving me a horrible headache. Now that I have discovered a magnificent nurse to care for me, I will see the dentist tomorrow," said Marx looking at Rachel. "I must warn you though; I am a very bad patient."

"It would be an honour," she answered with a smile. "Doctors make very bad patients I know. You should try to rest."

"I will be crying Chikuwaya, Chikuwaya and I won't allow you to leave my bed side," he said.

She burst out laughing, "I didn't know you were a very funny person. In my language, Chikuwaya means, it is paining."

***

Marx met Chola in theatre the next day. She had firmly resolved to have the amputation and even signed her own consent. Chola was sixteen and married. However, the theatre in-charge declined to accept her consent, citing that she was under age.

Marx entered theatre in his usual manner. He turned left and jumped into theatre Clogs.

There were four students he didn't recognize when he entered the duty room. Shifu and Johnny stood in the far right corner and leaned against a large old cabinet.

"Where are Jessica and Joan?" he asked.

"Dr Marximillian, we have four students from physiotherapy," the theatre nurse explained when she entered the duty room.

"I see," he remarked. "Have you ever witnessed an amputation?"

"Let them introduce themselves first," she said.

"I am Mutinta," said a tall young fellow standing next to Johnny.

"Annett," said a pretty and chubby girl. She sat on a chair opposite Marx on the large work table in the duty room.

"Melanie," a beautiful and shy young lady stated her name looking away from Marx. She sat on a bench just next to the door.

"My name is Yanika," said the last girl and smiled warmly. She had the most beautiful smile Marx had ever seen. He liked her immediately.

"Yanika," Marx repeated her name thoughtfully.

"It is a Dutch name," she said.

"Your name mm…meaning," he stated thoughtfully. "You have a strong need for freedom; physical, mental and spiritual. You hate bondage in any form. You are inventive, intuitive and extremely methodical. Since your will is so strong, you are hard to convince. You love beauty and philosophy, and you desire achievement."

"Doc," she said. "Is that what it means?"

"That is very true," Melanie agreed and let out a shy smile.

Marx had not met these wonderful physiotherapists. They were eager to witness an above elbow limb amputation. They sat in the duty room chatting with the medical students. They discussed theology, politics and love.

"Dr Marximillian, your patient has signed her own consent," the theatre nurse explained.

"And what is wrong with that?" he asked.

"She is under age. She is sixteen," she replied.

"She is married," said Yanika.

"That doesn't matter, I cannot allow her to come into my theatre," she answered.

"Sister, you don't want to start a fight with me. I have a terrible toothache right now. The last thing I want is you to be a pain in my neck. Give me the file, I will sign the damn consent," said Marx getting angry.

The nurse fled the duty room to find the file.

"Where are Jessica and Joan? They admitted her in casualty yesterday," said Marx standing up.

"We were there too, you have forgotten us doc," said Yanika with disappointment in her voice.

"Really, I am terribly sorry. Then tell us about her," he answered.

"She presented with a painful swollen crippled right hand and forearm of one week duration. She has history of being burnt in childhood at three months old. The burns involved her face, neck, chest and right upper limb. She has adduction contracture at the shoulder, flexion contracture at the elbow and hyper dorsi flexion at the wrist," Yanika gave a summary of Chola's affliction.

"Well done, I will send you to medical school," said Dr Marximillian visibly pleased with Yanika.

She smiled gorgeously at him. Just then, Joan and Jessica walked in with O'Neil and Ethel.

"Give us indications for Amputation?" he asked his students who had just walked in.

"Damn Nuisance Limb," O'Neil answered.

"Dying Limb," said Ethel.

"Dangerous Limb," said Joan.

"Dead Limb," Jessica answered.

"You are right, there are three broad indication for amputation of any body part, Dead, Deadly and Dead loss. Amputation is one of the oldest surgical procedures. Archaeologists have uncovered evidence of amputation; congenital or acquired through surgery or trauma in prehistoric humans. Upper extremity amputations largely follow the same basic principles as any other amputations," he explained.

"The patient is ready Dr Marximillian. Her mother signed the consent," the nurse announced.

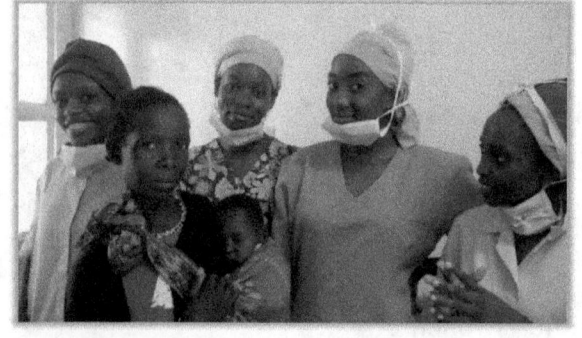

In the next twenty minutes, Chola lay on the operating table with a breathing tube protruding out of her mouth. The anaesthetist had chosen a general anaesthesia for this procedure. Dr Marximillian stood on the right of the operating table between Yanika and Jessica. Joan stood on Yanika's left. Shifu stood next to Jessica. Melanie and Annett lifted the mangled limb for Marx to clean. The girls looked beautiful in their theatre Regalia. Marx was delighted to have so many of them surrounding him.

As soon as he had finished cleaning the limb, he marked out his amputation line and cut deep through straps of biceps and Triceps. He quickly found the artery of the arm, the brachial artery and ligated it. He then searched for the three big nerves; the Median, Radial and Ulnar nerves. He passed Joan the surgical knife and asked her to cut the Radial nerve clean and high. He then gave Yanika to do the same with the Ulnar nerve. Jessica sliced through the Median nerve. The girls were ecstatic with their exploits.

"Nurse, pass the bone saw to Shifu, he is our bone surgeon," said Marx. His toothache had worsened and had a terrible headache as he worked.

Shifu positioned the saw and cut through the humerus after several back and forth strokes. Dr Marximillian reconstructed the stump and sent the patient to the ward.

His team was delight with the work they had done. They took photos with their patient in the recovery bay.

***

Dr Marximillian left theatre hastily to see the Dentist. He was just in time. He found him about to break off for lunch.

"Chikuwaya," he said pointing at his teeth.

The Dentist burst out laughing, "That is how my patients speak."

"I want it out my friend. This is the second attack I am having from the same tooth," Marx explained taking a seat on the massive dental chair.

"Let me take a look," said the dentist.

He inserted a shine, spoon like, round mirror into Marx's mouth and a wooden instrument to hold Dr Marximillian's tongue down.

"The tooth looks fine to me. I will just write you some antibiotics and you will be fine," he explained.

"No my friend, you have to pull it out. It is not fine, I feel it. I don't want to end up with a dental abscess and complicate into Ludwig's angina," Dr Marximillian protested.

"Doc, doc; you are thinking too much. Pulling a normal tooth can be dangerous. I may break it," the dentist tried to explain but Marx wouldn't take it.

"I can feel the nerve root is already involved," he insisted.

The poor dentist went back for a second look at his difficult patient's Premolar. He percussed all the teeth on the left side of the lower jaw. Each time he touched the rogue tooth, Marx screamed, Chikuwaya.

Reluctantly, the dentist agreed to pull it out. He injected Marx's gum with a local anaesthetic using the longest evil needle Marx had ever seen. It hurt so much and he cried Chikuwaya. He hadn't told the dentist he was hypertensive. When his gum became numb, his heart started to beat abnormally from the adrenaline in the anaesthetic. Dr Marximillian feared for his life.

The dentist searched his instrument kit and returned with an ugly looking thing. It looked like a pair of pliers used by carpenters to pull out stubborn nails. He grabbed Marx's rogue tooth and pulled on it. Marx felt a grating sound. He was afraid his tooth would shutter and disintegrate into multiple small fragments. His heart pounded and his face sweated profusely. He regretted making the decision. He wished his girls had escorted him. The tooth refused to give in no matter how much the dentist pulled.

The dentist pulled with all his strength but Marx's tooth refused to leave his mouth. When the local anaesthetic wore off, Marx realized he was now in serious trouble. He rose to spit the blood that had collected in his mouth. He couldn't believe what he saw. He was haemorrhaging profusely. The dentist looked scared. He realized he needed to encourage the poor fellow before he ended up being a referral.

"The tooth you are pulling has an abnormal anatomy. I had series of checks on it years ago. Don't worry it will come out. Just don't break my Jaw," he said laughing.

The dentist laughed. This talk helped him easy up. However, Marx feared he had got the wrong tooth. So he rose to examine himself in a mirror mounted over head. Satisfied it was the rogue tooth, he returned and slummed back into the dental chair. His heart was racing and he felt breathless. He took a deep breath and opened his mouth when the dentist had loaded a second cartridge into his dental gun. He drove his needle into Marx's palate and emptied its contents. It hurt so much prompting Marx to grab his hand and told him to wait. The adrenaline content was straining Dr Marximillian's heart.

The tooth only agreed to let go after an hour's struggle. The dentist agreed, it was the most difficulty extraction he had ever encountered. Marx remained in the chair fearing, he would pass out if he stood up.

After thirty minutes, his heart rate returned to normal and he could now stand. He thanked the dentist and left with his stubborn tooth wrapped in a piece of gauze and tucked away in his pocket. He decided to see Chola before leaving the hospital.

***

Dr Marximillian spent the evening wrestling the pain from his mouth. He had a fever and feared the dentist had pushed oral organisms into his blood stream. He was worried of developing sepsis. He considered calling the beautiful nurse Rachel to nurse him. He was certain, he needed intravenous antibiotics. The pain eased down by 9pm. He spat out the gauze the dentist had advised he bites on to stop him from haemorrhaging to death. He couldn't eat. He rinsed his mouth with an alcohol based mouth wash and felt much better.

He spent the night watching 'Gifted Hands', a movie the chief's daughter had given him. He couldn't stop being fascinated by Dr Ben Carson. He watched how a dumb and thick-headed black kid, with a violent temper, became the world's leading brain surgeon. The story of the German craniopagus twins could not cease to amuse Marx.

Patrick and Benjamin Binder were born in German on 2nd February, 1987. They were conjoined twins joined at the head. They were separated at John Hopkins Hospital on 7th September, 1987. They were the first twins to be successfully separated by a Neurosurgeon. That neurosurgeon was Ben Carson of Baltimore, Maryland.

Marx reflected on the outcome of that operation and what became of those boys as he lay nursing his wound. They were both left profoundly disabled. Two years after the separation, Patrick remained a vegetable. He never came out of his coma. Benjamin recovered to a certain extent. Their father was emotionally unable to ever handle them or share in their care. He became an alcoholic. Benjamin Binder never learned to speak or feed himself; however, he enjoys being taken for walks to this very day. **Patrick Binder died in his first decade of life. Their surgeon became a celebrity.**

Like many stories from the frontiers of medical science, it is a hard one to fit into an inspirational narrative, a tale of risk and loss and brutally tough Decisions. And although Dr Ben Carson and his team achieved something unprecedented, with long-term benefits for science, it did not result into a happily ever after story for the Binders. Their marriage fell apart.

Marx then reflected on current affairs. He focused his mind on American politics. Professor Dr Benjamin Carson had joined the presidential race on the republican ticket. But had since withdrawn from the race and endorsed the most unusual candidate the world had ever seen, Donald Trump. Many commentators likened him to Benito Andrea Mussolini and Adolf Hitler. Marx couldn't understand what had gone wrong with his mentor's brain, Dr Ben Carson. He couldn't understand why he chose to trade his operating theatre for a bruising race to the white house. He was sure; it was all about power and money. The good surgeon had fallen prey to the corrupting forces of Money and Power. He was certain Ben Carson's judgment had become clouded and inept on social matters. As if joining politics was not a decision bad enough, he shocked Marx when he endorsed Donald Trump for president of the United States.

"Who really owns doctors? Doctors are people too. Aren't they allowed to choose whatever career path in life to take? Even when that choice was supporting Donald Trump," he spoke loudly to his conscience. Marx couldn't hide the pain the choice his mentor had made caused him. He called it simply, Chikuwaya, a Chimambwe word for pain he had learnt in Mbala.

He turned his mind to think about Chola. He wondered how she was

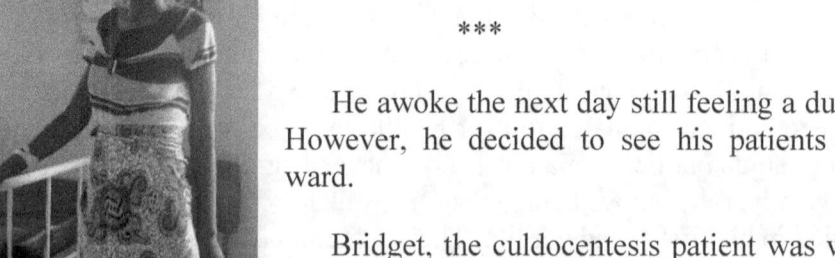

feeling on the cold open ward. If he couldn't stand just a tooth extraction, Chola must have been going through hell with an amputated arm.

***

He awoke the next day still feeling a dull ache. However, he decided to see his patients on the ward.

Bridget, the culdocentesis patient was walking now and feeding normally. She was delighted to see Dr Marximillian that morning. He took photos with her. She made him forgot about his aching gum and headache. She sat on a bed his earlier patient, Rhoda, had not risen from. She had been moved to the gynecology ward owing to her three week old baby. Marx wondered how Rhoda was in Kasama. No one on the ward expected Bridget to live. They were amazed at how she had recovered. Many in the hospital and patients on the ward begun to believe, Dr Marximillian's touch could heal a sick patient. They were convinced God's favour was upon his life. However, they were unaware about the struggles he had in his personal life. His amazing practice was under serious threat from evil people that had conspired to take away his salary. He was convinced; this would probably be his last practice.

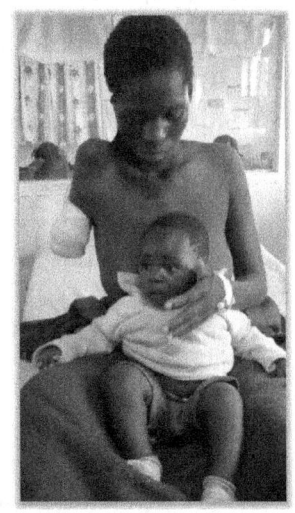

Chola spent an uneventful night. She was smiling when she saw her doctor. She thanked him for taking away the mangled limb that had troubled her for sixteen years. He found her holding her baby.

"Uli Chola?" Dr Marximillian greeted her.

"Ningo sili, ya doctor," she answered.

"How is the wound?" he asked.

"Chikuwaya panono," she answered.

Like many of his patients, Chola was from an island on Lake Tanganyika. Marx worried how she was going to manage with one limb. He wished he could find her an upper limb prosthesis. The girls from physiotherapy had talked about starting a foundation called, 'Help Chola International', to raise funds for Chola's prosthesis and help make cooking environments safe for children on the island where Chola was burnt.

Chola's husband was around when Marx went to see her. He had arrived from Mpulungu. He was in his early twenties. He was disheveled and wore a dirty over coat. It was cold in Mbala. However, he was a cheerful young fellow. Marx liked him immediately.

***

Later that night, Marx found himself wrestling the Mbala winter. He couldn't feel his own feet. He was sure his room had turned into a freezer. His blankets could not keep him warm. He found himself texting the girls about the harsh winter he was experiencing in his room.

"I am freezing guys, I need the King's formula," he sent a wechat text to his girls.

"Cup of really hot tea works well," Yanika replied almost immediately.

"Only the King's formula can work in Mbala winter," he insisted.

"kkkkk, Mbala winter," Yanika wechated back

"What is the King's formula?" Joan asked.

"When King David was old and well advanced in years, he could not keep warm even when they put covers over him. So his servants said to him, 'let us look for a young virgin to attend the king and take care of him. She can lie beside him so that our lord the king may keep warm'; 1 Kings 1:1," Marx sprinkled scripture on his bait.

"What was her name? I am sure she was hot…lol," Joan replied walking into the lure.

"What was her name?" Jessica asked curiously.

"…if two lie down together, they will keep warm. But how can one keep warm alone? Eccl 4:11;" Yanika sugar coated the lure.

"Who will choose for you?" Melanie asked.

"We will use the King's Formula," Marx reset the decoy.

"How did they do it?" Jessica.

"They searched throughout Israel for a beautiful girl and found Abishag, a Shunammite, and brought her to the king. The girl was very beautiful; she took care of the king…," he wrote quoting 1Kings 1:3-4

"I have already chosen for you," Yanika replied.

"Kkkkk, I know her," Joan responded promptly.

"Hhhhhh," Selym laughed suspiciously.

"Pwapwapwa….. Hope not a local girl from Mpulungu," read Annett's text.

"I miss you personally," a text came on a number he had not saved in his phone book.

He diagnosed the author of the unanimous text to be suffering from *MOSS*, Multi Orifice Starvation Syndrome, a debilitating illness aggravated by the Mbala winter.

"Let me chose for you," Melanie offered to help.

"Doc, about femur fractures, should we continue placing blocks on the bed to support the fracture site," Annett asked changing the subject.

"Accurate opposition and rigid immobilization are not essential for femoral shaft fractures but traction is required to prevent overlap," he replied.

The girls were prolific short hand text writers. Marx found he could not keep up with the traffic of texts reaching his phone. He fell asleep leaving a string of unanswered texts.

Some Trails are Happy Ones

Dr Marximillian began his last week in Mbala in the usual way. He conducted his ward rounds, completed his theatre lists and attended out patients clinics.

He lay in bed on his last Wednesday morning reminiscing what an incredible vacation he had to Mbala. This was his nineteenth day; he was scheduled to leave on Day Twenty One, that same week over the weekend. He was pleased with the work he had done. The average temperature was set at 18.2 degrees. He had been totally won over by this weather and had buried himself into what he loved most, his work. The Charity that had promised to finance his medical retreat did not honor its word. He was bankrupt; however he was pleased he had been able to be of service to the poor of Abercorn community.

***

At the hospital, Chola was doing very well. Rachel had changed the dressing and was looking forward to a generous compliment from Dr Marximillian. In gynecology ward, Bridget was back from the grave. She had cheated death in full view of everyone. Dr Marximillian felt he was wrongly credited for her resurrection. He was glad; his God had not left him after all.

He arrived at the car park in a Taxi belonging to his Ten Kwacha Mbala entrepreneur driver. He disembarked and hurried for the wards. The giant Miombo and Acacia Albina trees performed a Mexican wave as he walked towards the wide foot path close by. On his left, he passed an old Vitex Doniana tree, which the locals called Umucinka. He met O'Neil and

Ethel in the wide corridor leading from the outpatient department. They informed him the patients were stable.

On hearing this, Marx decided to visit the old hospital. His busy schedule had prevented him from visiting this section of Abercorn community Hospital. This fragment of the hospital had served the white settlers in the pre independence era, now it lay in ruins.

Marx pondered over what really constituted a good hospital. Marx was convinced, as Linda, a good hospital wasn't one made out of great brick walls; but one made out of a motivated, well remunerated and dedicated professional team of health workers. He believed hospitals were dichotomous. Composed of static structures and a fluid facet; the dynamic human elements that made up the functional unit of the hospital.

Walls never remember those who walk passed them. The historical

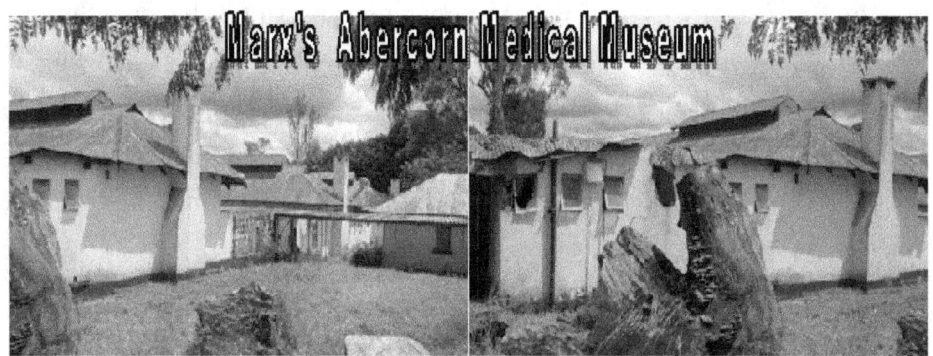

walls Marx was admiring had no memory or knowledge of care. He wished they could tell him about the vibrant staff that once served there; the gossips they shared behind the walls and the sick they looked after.

The dilapidated walls merely stared at him as he passed through history. However, he was aware they once offered an excellent aesthetic element to the complex mosaic of health delivery in Abercorn. He wondered at how many people were still alive that had worked there or been admitted to the desolate wards. The corridors upon which he walked once hosted a lively health care team of ambitious colleagues and compassionate nurses and doctors. Marx wondered how they would feel if they returned to their old work place. He was certain the hospital walls would make them feel like they were visiting a cemetery or a museum. There own sight would be fading and failing; and would not be able to recognize what Marx was admiring.

Like Linda, the dichotomy of every hospital greatly fascinated Marx. He wondered how it would be to have a model fluid hospital that grew and aged with the community it saved. He was looking at a piece of Art, that only the wise could appreciate and enjoy. In his mind's eye, he could see the forbearers of the great work of medicine in Abercorn going about their day to day duties. He was delighted to have been privileged to walk in their footsteps.

Marx made a right turn at the far end of the corridor and walked a few paces from there. This route led him to a wide open section. There were several buildings in Victorian architecture and countless tree species, indigenous and exotic. Marx stood in awe, admiring several chalets from the bygone era. Several giant trees had been brutally cut down by humans who didn't value history. There were large fallen tree trunks everywhere he looked. He spotted Umufungo, a tree valued for its fruits, firewood and medicinal properties. A few paces from where he stood, he saw several Galcinia species, known locally as Umusoko. This tree was valuable to

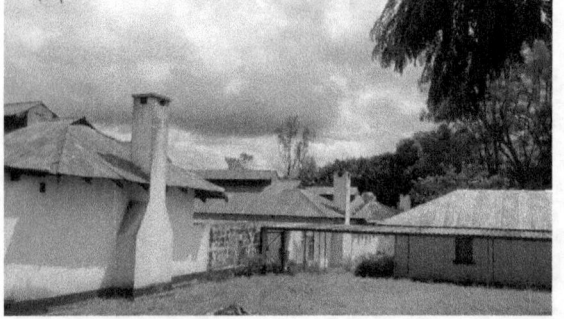

fruit eating birds in the area. Humans used Umusoko for fiber and for making Poles. He walked like a botanist fascinated by the old trees he saw. He came to an old Acacia Albina tree next to a beautiful Chalet. Locally, this tree was known as Umungamununsi and birds loved to nest in its branches. Several birds perched in its branches as he passed. He saw two doves grooming each other. They were deeply in love. He tried to search for their nest but decided not to disturb these love birds. He moved on to another tree nearby.

Marx stood under an old Umuula tree (*parinari curatelliofolia*) reflecting how life must have been in this Garden of Eden. He thought it was the most beautiful place he had ever seen. Old giant Jacaranda trees stood inter spaced with the old buildings. Beautiful Large chimneys could be seen on all the buildings. They projected from the walls and towered above the old buildings elegantly. They stood as testimony to the blistering cold that pounded Mbala. At their peak, they had protected the patients and staff from the notorious Mbala winter. Dr Marximillian wished the community could find a curator to care for this fascinating area.

Marx was cognizant of the fact that, he had just walked through an icon of medical history in Mbala. He wished this area could be turned into a museum.

In one of the Chalets he passed, he found a beautiful ante natal mother. She had travelled from her village of Nsokolo, to seek a safe delivery at ACH. Marx was curious to enter one of these chalets and admire the interior.

This complex Marx explored was known as the mother's shelter. Several other people from outside Mbala used it as a place of refuge while waiting for their sick relatives on the ward.

The chalet Marx chose offered basic living conditions for the ante natal mother. It was her first pregnancy. She shared this hut with four other elderly women who had travelled with her. They welcomed Dr Marximillian to their humble dwelling. They smiled warmly at him and invited him to join them for lunch. He thanked them but declined to rob them of their food.

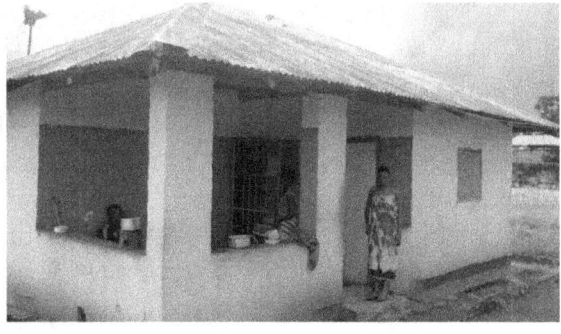

The chalet was divided into two areas; a lounge and a sleeping area. It had no running water. There were no beds to be found. There was one mattress on the floor, an old mosquito net hang over it. Marx figured this was for the expectant mom. The other women had their beddings rolled out and heaped in one corner. The lounge area had no seats; the elderly ladies used it as their kitchen.

Marx left the chalet, after thanking the occupants, to explore a little further. He ran into a man just winding his lunch. He told Marx his wife, a Tanzanian national, was admitted to the hospital. He was there to wait for her. The couple lived in Mtula, in Tanzania.

Marx didn't like his living quarters. An old mattress, he called his bed was placed on the floor in one corner. His beddings were folded and placed in a red bag in the other corner next to his faithful

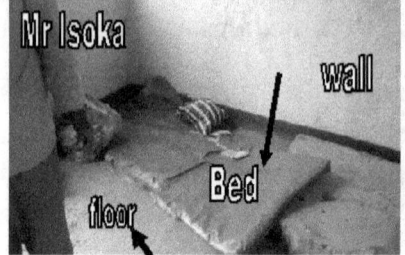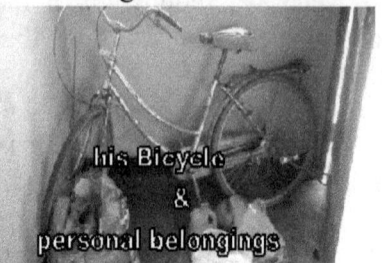

old bicycle. He was a very cheerful man. He never complained about his predicaments. However, he was deeply worried about his wife's failing health.

While Marx chatted with Mr. Isoka, his phone rang; it was Yanika. The girls wanted him to join them for Lunch. He bade Mr. Isoka farewell and wished his wife quick recovery.

***

Yanika had come with Melanie to fetch Marx. They looked beautiful in their white shirts and navy blue trousers. Their beautiful trousers angled benevolently at the hip. The shirts were, sometimes, cut short to allow the hip to stand out. The final result, made the girls look like models. Marx thought they had deliberately tempered with their trousers at the waist to give this dazzling effect.

He followed the beautiful girls to their hostel. They passed an old garden with several fruit trees. Large old tree trunks lay about against unattended green bushes in the garden. Marx wondered why these trees had been cruelly cut. He wished he could carbon date these trees.

"We saw Chola today, she looks beautiful," said Melanie walking leisurely, enjoying Dr Marximillian's towering presence.

"Yes, and we saw her cute baby boy," Yanika remarked. "And she is only sixteen."

"I haven't been to the wards today, I decided to give myself a tour of the old hospital," said Marx following his pretty captors.

"She looks older than sixteen," said Yanika.

"She is truly sixteen. Her mother remembers her birthday vividly and even the day she got burnt," said Melanie. She looked up at Marx who was walking between the girls.

They came to an open space were they found several other students Marx had not met. They were doing their laundry. Shifu, Joan and Johnny were among the students Marx recognized. Their hostels looked dilapidated, however the students looked cheerful. They were delighted to see Dr Marximillian visiting their compound.

"Welcome doc," Johnny called out. "This is where we live."

Marx waved at the students. He knew in his heart, these were Zambia's next generation of Doctors and health care professionals. There were no washing machines in the hostels. They washed their cloths with bare hands. He wondered what impact this dilapidated dwelling would have on their future practice of medicine. He hoped his time with some of them had positively impacted their future practice. He was proud; his desires of the flesh had not taken advantage of his beautiful students. He was a proud man as he strolled through

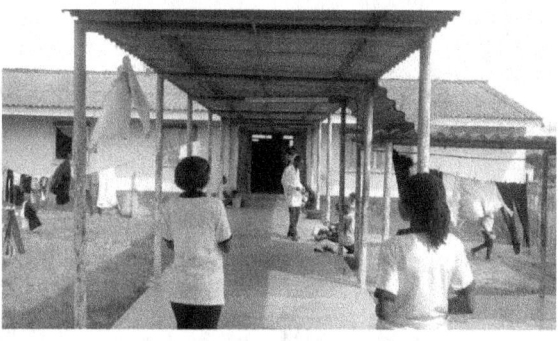

their living quarters. Everyone thought he was an upright man; it was a generous view he did not share.

Joan had a large pile of laundry in a yellow bucket opposite to where Marx stood to greet the students. She was scrubbing her slippers when Marx passed by. She greeted him and smiled gorgeously at him. Marx loved this girl. He was convinced with proper training and right mentorship, she could make a great surgeon. She had great hands for surgery. He admired her long fingers that were busy scrubbing slippers as he passed by.

His hosts took him on a quick tour of their rooms. They were humble living quarters. Yanika shared a small bed with Melanie. The room was small and neatly arranged. It smelled a sweet feminine aroma. The light was dim and offered a perfect place to cure Insomnia and *MOSS*.

"You have a beautiful house," he said standing in the middle of the room.

"Thank you doc," said Yanika. "I share it with Melanie. Even at school we are roommates."

They walked to a third room where the food was set. There were several rooms on either side of this long corridor they passed through.

"Who else lives here," he asked looking at the long narrow corridor they were walking through. The walls were painted blue and looked clean.

"Nurses and other workers from the hospital," Melanie answered.

"We were lucky to have been allocated these rooms in this block. Usually students are not allocated here," said Yanika turning into a room radiating a sweet aroma.

No sooner did he enter than Marx's mouth begun to water. He was hungry.

"What is this place?" he asked.

"Welcome to our Kitchen doc," said Yanika showing him a seat.

"We wanted to give you a farewell luncheon," said Annett.

"The food smells so sweet, not only are you beautiful, you are good cooks too. Thank you for inviting me," he said seating down.

A handsome young man sat on the bed. He was busy on his computer when they walked in.

"That is Mutinta, he is our young brother," said Yanika introducing the handsome young man on the bed.

"Welcome doc," he said warmly.

"You are one blessed fellow. All these beautiful sisters taking care of you; you must be in heaven," said Marx smiling.

"This is our physiotherapy team. We were posted the four of us and we are classmates back at school," said Yanika. She looked like the group's leader.

"I hope you have room for one more, because I am joining this progressive team with immediate effect," said Marx.

The girls burst out laughing.

"So, tell me about yourselves," he asked.

Annett put the food on the bed, "Forgive us doc, our bed is also our dining table."

"Don't worry about me, I can even dine from the floor, you have a lovely place here," he answered.

The girls served Nshima with sausage and vegetables. And a special dish of soya beans, which they called 'chunks'. Dr Marximillian enjoyed their food profoundly. He loved this wonderful family. Marx found all his desires of the flesh left him at once. He could no longer think of eloping with anyone of them.

He told them about a restaurant in town where he ran away at the site of the food he had ordered.

"I was so hungry… when the waiter returned with my order, I fled. She must have thought I had seen a ghost," he told them. They burst out laughing at him. "Until that day, I had never seen such frightening plate of Nshima and fish before."

"Doc, you are killing me," Melanie protested. She was laughing continuously looking at Marx.

Annett stood up and offered Marx a cup of water. He got it from her and thanked her sincerely.

"Yanika, where is home?" Marx asked seeing she had become quiet.

"I come from Mulenga Hills, overlooking Soft Katongo. My grandparents live on the edge of a large mountain called Mulenga," she said and smiled warmly at him.

"The man I was talking to when you called me, he attended Soft Katongo primary school. He is from Isoka but he lives in Tanzania," said

Marx thinking about Mr. Isoka. "He is nursing his wife in the hospital. They came cycling from Mtula in Tanzania."

"Mutinta is from Monze but he has never lived there," said Annett laughing. "I am from Zambezi."

Mutinta smiled quietly, "That's true, I have never been to Monze doc."

He was a very quiet fellow. He spoke very little. The girls loved him like a brother.

"Melanie is from Njola Mwanza," said Yanika.

"My Grand Mother lives in Njola, in Monze," said Melanie.

"You could be my cousin; my mother is from Njola," Marx smiled at Melanie.

"Really," she smiled adorably at him.

"Did you know…, *Gone with the Wind* inspired a generation of girls named Melanie. It was the name of two Roman saints of the fifth century, a grandmother and granddaughter. The name was introduced to England from France in the Middle Ages. In the US, Melanie became a Top 100 name in the late sixties, and remains still at number 80," said Marx looking at Melanie.

"Wow, I love it… I didn't know that," said Melanie admiring Marx visibly.

"No wonder, you are a doc, you know too many things," said Yanika smiling. "Doesn't your head feel heavy sometimes? I am sure you experience migraines a lot."

"He is like Google search engine, he never sleeps," remarked Mutinta who had been quiet all this while.

After a scrumptious meal in the students' hostel, they left for the hospital. Marx was grateful the girls had arranged a surprise and wonderful farewell luncheon for him.

The laundry area that had buzzed with numerous students was quiet now. They had all returned to the hospital. Their cloths hung on the lines and some where spread on the grass and bushes in the compound and fallen tree trunks. Nostalgic memories of his own student days hit him as they passed the hostel square. He walked with Mutinta, Melanie and Annett on the wide corridor leading to the exit.

Yanika had remained behind to tidy up. Marx turned and walked back to wait for her. He loved this young lady. He found her intelligent, pretty and beautiful and she had gorgeous legs. Since the desires of his flesh had left him, he couldn't harbour selfish desires after her. It was raining outside. The temperature had plummeted. Marx was freezing, however he no longer longed for the King's formula.

Yanika emerged skipping as she walked. She looked gorgeous.

"You came back for me," she said when she saw him.

"Yes," he answered. "I thought you would get lost."

She smiled, and walked silently towards him. Had it been in the movies, she would have walked straight at him and thrown herself in his big surgical arms and given him a deep good bye kiss.

"I wanted to take you to Munada. I wish you would still be around," she said.

"What is Munada?" he asked walking beside her.

"Munada is Swahili for open market; it is a kind of fair held on the 4th and 15th of every month in old location. It brings together local small scale business people in Zambia and Tanzania. You would love it," she said skipping with an imaginary rope in front of him.

"I like your legs," he said looking at her.

"They are too big," she giggled and turned around to face him.

"They are strong and gorgeous," he insisted.

"Thank you," she answered calmly. "No one has ever told me such kind words before."

They caught up with the rest of the team in the corridor going down to outpatient. The Team bade farewell when they reached a right turn leading to maternity and surgical wards.

The rains had engulfed ACH. Several people stood along the corridors to shelter from the rains. The car park was transformed into numerous pools of water. The rains showed no signs of letting off any time soon. It was cold. Several people; hospital staff, patients and their relatives stood in clusters all along the corridor. Many had their hands tucked under their armpits to keep warm. Marx stood enjoying the serenity brought by the cold and these torrential rains. He could forgive a cliché forming in his mind. " All is well that ends well," he thought.

***

Later that evening, Marx sat in his Room at Giza. He reflected on his stay in Mbala and smiled to himself. He still had one thing left to do, a visit to the local Museum. He planned on taking Yanika's family with him the following day. He had heard rumor about an eerie section in the museum that specialized in magic and traditional medicine.

He wanted to see the Inkuwa, a notorious charm used to strike lightening. There were other creepy charms he had been told about. He meticulously jotted down the names he had been told; Sinsimwi, a charm for causing misery and death. Lukulo, a charm used for stealing other people's items. Mwanzabamba wa nsoka, a charm for sending snakes to attack victims. Kalowe Noko, a charm for sending ghosts. Buta, a charm used to suck blood from victims. Umukana, a charm used to cause instability in homes. Ignini, a kind of traditional landmine believed to kill those who pass over it. Insunsi also known as Longalonga, a charm used to cause pain and death. And finally; Akambuma, a charm used to steal other people's items. He felt his hair stand on end as he jotted down these spooky charms. He couldn't wait to see this collection of man's wicked heart.

He couldn't bring himself to imagine the evil face of a man who had power to send his fellow man a100 million volts wrapped in a bolt of lightning.

Now, lightening is sudden electrostatic discharge during an electrical storm between electrically charged regions of a cloud. There were three types of lightening Marx knew; IC, CC and CG for Intra- cloud lightning, between one cloud and another cloud lightning and between a cloud and the ground lightning respectively. There was a fourth the physicists did not know about. The man made lightning of Mbala. Probably the Intra- Cloud, IC, lightning was Inkuwa after all.

Dr Marximillian was much more interested to check out the Traditional Medicines section. He had studied Medicinal chemistry and couldn't wait to lay his hands on some raw materials for testing in his home based laboratory. He had heard about Akamyanshinge, a potent Aphrodisiac for treating impotence in men and that could arouse incredible libido in both sexes. He had also heard about Musengele, a potent love charm. Marx also hoped to lay his hands on Kaselelele, a potent traditional Oxytocic drug used to accelerate labour in home deliveries and probably responsible for some of the uterine raptures he had attended at ACH. The Moto Moto museum was a Must see for Dr Marximillian. He couldn't wait to experiment with a pinch of Musengele on lady Yanika and Melanie.

As he thought these things, his phone rang. It was the coverage nurse. There was an emergency at the hospital and they wanted him urgently.

"Doc, I have a woman with Hb 6g/dl. She has APH at term. I can't appreciate the foetal heart beat. She is only a tip of finger and she is 'O' minus. There is no blood in the hospital. I am considering referring her," the doctor on call explained.

"Let me come over," Dr Marximillian replied.

The emergency vehicle arrived shortly. It was 11 pm in Mbala. They drove for the hospital immediately. The driver was counting on Marx to call off the referral to Kasama, and save him 400 km night driving. They drove in the dark silently. It was late and Marx was tired. He summoned his mind to recall all what he knew about APH.

Now APH is Antepartum Haemorrhage or heavy bleeding before delivery. This call brought a deluge of nostalgic memories of Marx's days as an OBGY Resident. The Landcruiser bounced and jerked on the treacherous bumpy gravel road to the Hospital. It was dark all around except for the poor light from the head lumps and tail lights of the old cruiser. It was cold inside the cruiser. Its wipers worked frantically to keep an unrelenting drizzle over Mbala off its cracked windscreen. Visibility was poor. Dr Marximillian was glad it was only a short drive to the hospital.

On arrival at the hospital, Marx rushed to the Maternity ward through the dark corridors. He found the Doctor on call anxiously waiting for him as where several midwives on duty. His students had gone to the ward too when news about this emergency reached them.

"Hi guys," he greeted the students in his usual calm temperament. "What do you have doc."

"I think we should just refer this woman doc," the exhausted doctor on call gave his opinion. He had surrendered.

"Do you think she has better chance of survival if you refer her than here? Remember Kasama is not next door," Dr Marximillian challenged the poor doctor.

"Her Hb is 6g/dl and we have no blood in the hospital," a midwife came to the rescue of the doctor.

Marx turned to his students and begun to teach.

"Obstetric haemorrhage remains one of the major causes of maternal death in developing countries. The causes of APH include; Placenta previa, Placental abruption and local causes. It is not uncommon to fail to identify a cause of APH, when it is then described as 'unexplained APH'.

"I was thinking she has a ruptured uterus or placenta previa," the doctor on call tried to explain.

"No doc, this is Placental abruption," Dr Marximillian explained walking over to the patient.

"How can you tell placenta previa from placenta abruption," O'Neil asked.

"Usually placenta previa causes painless bleeding," Joan answered.

"That is very correct Dr Joan. Abruptio placentae is defined as the premature separation of a normally positioned placenta from the wall of the uterus, usually after 20 weeks of pregnancy. Patients with Abruptio placentae, also called placental abruption, typically present with vaginal bleeding, painful uterine contractions, and fetal distress or death like in our case here," Dr Marximillian explained.

While Marx taught, he was worried his patient might develop the most feared complication of all; couvelaire's uterus. This was his last week in

Mbala and the last thing he needed was a patient dying on the operating table. He knew everyone would forget all the good surgeries he had performed and only remember this one poor outcome. He stood for a while and pondered the words of the doctor on call to refer the patient to die on the way to Kasama. He was almost certain; this was a conspiracy against the good work he had done. The temptation to refer the patient weighed heavily on his mind.

"Are you going to operate with Hb of 6 or allow her to deliver vaginally since the baby is dead?" Jessica asked looking very worried and concerned for the poor patient.

"The cervix is only admitting a tip of finger. Vaginal delivery is the best choice with a non viable fetus. However, our patient will exsanguinate before we could achieve that. Even then, she would be at risk of PPH from couvelaire's uterus. And complicate into or die from Disseminated Intravascular Coagulopathy and Acute Renal Failure," Dr Marximillian laid out his worst case scenario.

"What is Couvelaire's uterus and DIC?" Joan asked with a *Marximused* look on her face.

"Couvelaire's uterus my dear, also known as uteroplacental apoplexy, is a life threatening condition in which loosing of the placenta, Abruptio placentae, causes bleeding that penetrates into the uterine muscles , the myometrium, forcing its way into the peritoneal cavity. The treatment involves immediate evacuation of the uterus and stimulating uterine contractions with intravenous oxytocin; Hysterectomy, the removal of the uterus, may be needed in some cases," Dr Marximillian explained to his stunned team. "DIC is a serious disorder in which the proteins that control blood clotting become over active.

"Hysterectomy with Hb of 6; doc let us just refer this patient to Kasama. She will die on us. I don't want her blood on my hands," the doctor on call reiterated his call for referral.

"I think Dr Ibu is right. Let us just refer her. We have no blood here," the Midwife answered taking Dr Ibu side.

"Those in favour of referral raise your hands," Mr. Ibu and the midwife raised their hands. "If Medicine was a democracy, we would have settled this by a show of hands. Fortunately it is not. This is why I think our current voting system, one man one vote, is foolish;. You and I have the same voting power as a retarded unschooled bastard who spends his day drinking at a street corner somewhere. I think each of your votes should equal a thousand votes," he said

"Your vote Dr Marximillian should equal a million votes," said Joan smiling.

"I couldn't agree with you more my love," he answered smiling warmly at Joan. "I called Kasama on my way here. They have no blood. It would be tantamount to immorality to send this patient a long way off, only to die on the way to Kasama. This might be her only window of survival. If she must die by my hand, so be it. Sister, prepare this patient for surgery; we are going in. Girls, you will be my assistant surgeons.

"Doc, this patient was in shock when I was called. Her uterus was not contracting that is why I thought she had placenta previa. She may truly have couvelaire's uterus. The uterus won't contract. You may truly be faced with a hysterectomy with an Hb of 6. I have never seen anyone perform a hysterectomy under these circumstances. I have a feeling this is not likely to turn out right," Dr Ibu spelt out his consternation.

"May be this is her appointed time to die. Why can't you just leave her alone to die peacefully? I have a bad feeling about this too," the midwife echoed Dr Ibu's premonition.

"I am a scientist. I do not use feelings. I make scientific decisions," Dr Marximillian put his foot down.

Everyone was quiet. The students brought the theatre trolley. The anesthetist watched quietly at a distance. He knew Marx would not walk away from the patient even when her chances of survival were bleak.

(Medical Jargon below [*in italics*], may skip without loss to story flow)

"For my baby doctors, I want to tell you a little bit about the pathophysiology of this killer condition. Like I said earlier; *Couvelaire's uterus is a phenomenon wherein the retro-placental blood may penetrate through the thickness of the wall of the uterus into the peritoneal cavity. This may occur after Abruptio placentae. The hemorrhage that gets into the deciduas basalis ultimately splits the decidua, and the hematoma may remain within the decidua or may extravasate into the myometrium. The myometrium becomes weakened and may rupture due to the increase in intrauterine pressure associated with uterine contractions,"* he explained. *"Whereas, Disseminated Intravascular Coagulopathy is characterized by systemic activation of blood coagulation, which results in generation of and deposition of fibrin, leading to micro vascular thrombi in various organs and contributing to multiple organ dysfunction syndrome. Consumption and subsequent exhaustion of clotting factors or coagulation proteins and platelets, from ongoing activation of coagulation, may induce severe bleeding. Therefore, we define DIC as an acquired syndrome characterized by the intravascular activation of coagulation with loss of localization arising from different causes."*

"This patient is already showing signs of DIC and he insists on going ahead with surgery," Dr Ibu whispered to the midwife. Marx overheard their gossip.

"I heard that," he answered. "God did not send me here to slaughter his people. He promised to save everyone I touched. I believe he is with us right now. This is not a feeling. It is scientifically true. I have evidence he has been with me since I came here as he has been with me in my practice back in my hospital. Do you know where David drew the courage to slay the giant?"

"From God," Jessica answered.

"It is written in 1 Samuel 17:32-37," Marx decided to quote his favourite scriptures;

> David said to Saul, "Let no one lose heart on account of this Philistine; your servant will go and fight him."

> Saul replied, "You are not able to go out against this philistine and fight him; you are only a boy and he has been a warrior from his youth."

> But David said to Saul, "Your servant has been keeping his father's sheep. When a lion or bear came and carried off a sheep from the flock, I went after it, struck it and rescued the sheep from its mouth. When it turned on me, I seized it by its hair, struck it and killed it. Your servant has killed both the lion and the bear; this uncircumcised Philistine will be like one of them, because he has defied the armies of the living God. The LORD who rescued me from

the paw of the lion and the paw of the bear will rescue me from the hand of this Philistine."

The team arrived in theatre. The patient was laid on the table. Dr Marximillian instructed his young doctors to scrub in and assist him.

"No, I will assist," Dr Ibu protested. "I have heard about your bullet speed surgeries. I would like to witness one with my own naked eyes."

"Be my guest doubting Thomas," Marx replied and grinned at the girls.

Dr Marximillian and Dr Ibu scrubbed in the usual way. They then approached the theatre nurse on her instruments table. She gowned them in the usual elaborate etiquette of the operating theatre. Soon they were standing on the operating table ready to start the surgery. Doubt was written all over Dr Ibu's face. Marx chose to ignore his facial expressions.

He opened the patient's abdomen using a lower bikini line incision. Within seconds he delivered the dead baby before Dr Ibu could say couvelaire's uterus. He passed it to the equally *Marximused* midwife still attached to its placenta. He then turned his attention to the uterus as Dr Ibu's hands trembled continuously. Marx was certain his assistant would suffer a syncope attack and faint on him.

"Are you ok doc?" Marx asked him.

"You are a magician doc," he answered fumbling for words. "I have never witness such speed in my entire practice of medicine. I thought people were exaggerating when they talked about you. Now I have seen for myself. You are incredible doc."

While Dr Ibu stood dazed by the rapidly changing operating techniques he was witnessing, Dr Marximillian had completed detaching the uterus from its upper attachments and pedicles. He spared both ovaries after examining them meticulously. The patient hardly bled.

"Where did you learn all this," the *Marximused* Dr Ibu asked. "I should have known. I wouldn't have talked about that referral. I would have just sent for you immediately."

"I learned it as a shepherd boy tending my sheep in remote local brown pastures," he replied placing clamps on utero- sacral ligaments. "We need to suture the vaginal vault to these ligaments to prevent prolapsed in the future."

"Hysterectomy in twelve minutes, I must be dreaming," Dr Ibu remarked utterly *Marximesmerized*.

"It is not a dream doc," the anesthetist answered him. "This is why I have always been telling you to tag along and learn before this man goes back to his hospital. This is how he works. It is like magic."

"I take off my hat for you," said Dr Ibu bowing down.

"Igue," Marx answered bowing down too.

Meantime, Joan, Jessica and Selym followed the midwife to take a close look at the dead baby. The boys, Johnny, O'Neil and Shifu took the couvelaire's uterus to the sluice room for closer examination. By now, Marx had placed five sutures on the patient's abdomen and the theatre nurse was preparing a dressing for the wound. The anesthetist instituted his steps for reversal of his patient from anesthesia. It was a successful operation. One still talked about at ACH to this very day.

***

Back in his room at Giza, he thought about the chief's daughter and decided to text her. She was in Kitwe.

"Isabelle, this is my 19th day in your beautiful town. I will be leaving in two days," he wrote.

"21 days already; I wish I was there to say goodbye. It is not fair," she wrote back almost immediately.

"Bye bye, you are the sweetest friend I ever had in Mbala," he replied

"I'll miss you terribly. I am so lonely. How can the two people that made me smile in the same week go at the same time," she protested.

"You are in Kitwe, how can you be lonely? Keep smiling," he replied.

"I am not smiling nicely right now, you know," she sent him a sad face emoticon.

"Laughter is a medicine. I prescribe smiles for you and laughter eight times a day," he tried to cheer her.

"Kkkkk; I will live to remember you for the rest of my life as a man who never took advantage of me even when I was so close to him," she sent him a blushing Emoticon.

"Wow, thank you very much. There is a Ghanaian saying; 'a man who keeps a beautiful lady for a friend is like a person who keeps a Guinea Fowl for a pet. He is likely to eat his poor pet one day," he sent her a warning wrapped in an African proverb.

"Kkkkk; provided he is an excellent cook, it is fine," she replied in her usual unpredictable naughty trait.

"I am so glad I never took advantage of you. Did you know I thought of turning you into a Braii pack many times in Mpulungu? Thank you for helping me not to. You are an incredible young lady. You are funny and naughty. I will miss you daily," he thanked her for their memorable retreat to Mpulungu.

"I was vulnerable, I wanted you… but you chose not to take advantage of me. Thank you for inspiring me to see beyond the moment. You are a good man, a compassionate doctor and a gifted surgeon. I will always cherish my memories of you working late in the night on the wards and as a fish expert of Lake Tanganyika. You will always be, for me, a giant among a few good doctors," she summarized how she would remember Marx.

"These are the sweetest words I have ever heard," he expressed his sincere appreciation of her kind words.

"I am serious…," she texted him back immediately.

"If you are ever in the Tourist Capital my Lady, you remain forever my adorable Princess and I, a friend you can truly trust forever," he replied.

***

THE END

Also by Dr K C Moonga

1. *Finding Linda*

   (Book about Mysterious encounters in the hospital)
2. *The Missing Link*

   (Cancer Awareness book based on true life accounts)

3. *I Know What You Did in China*

4. *Girl Child Menstrual Care & GBV awareness Book*

5. *First Lady's Menstrual Care & GBV awareness Book*

6. *A Few Good Doctors*

7. *The Practice*

You can get all books Online. Visit amazon.com or contact Dr Kelvin C Moonga on drkmoonga2011@live.com; drkmoonga2011@gmail.com

Wechat and WatsApp # +260965868668

www.amazon.com

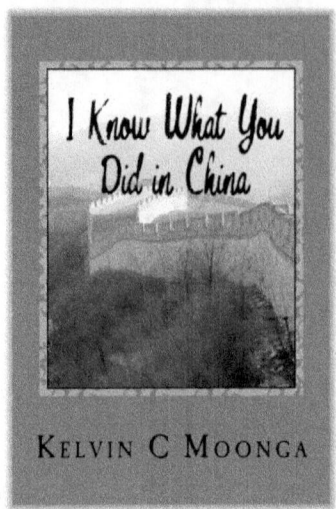

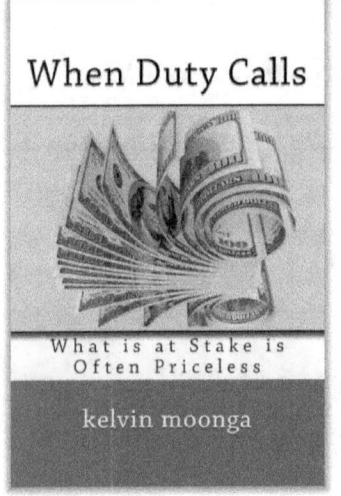

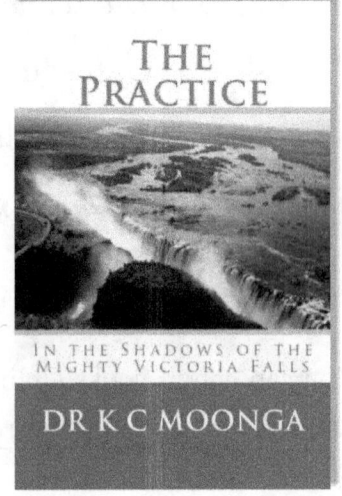

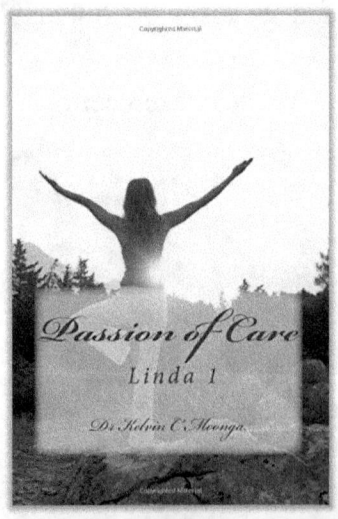

The Menstrual Cycle is the most amazing phenomenon in the life of a woman. Its beginning, referred to as Menarche, announces monumental changes in the life of a girl child. Its end, referred to as Menopause, ushers in other monumental changes in the lives of many women. Some of these changes are so intense that they can alter a woman's personality. This can affect her social functioning beginning at home, school and work places.

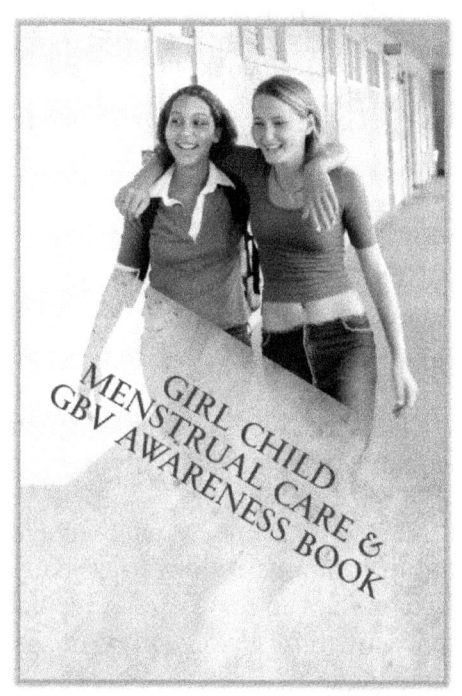

The Adolescent Girl Child needs special education to understand the hormonal storm raging inside her young and naive body. Everyone expects her to hurriedly learn to manage herself and navigate the complex world around her. She is often judged harshly when she stumbles and Falls.

The menstrual cycle causes her to lose blood every Month. This may cause her Anemia, a medical condition that is characterized by; poor concentration, headaches, dizziness, weakness, getting tired easily, reduced mental capacity, low immunity, poor wound healing, poor appetite, lethargy, fainting, heart failure, poor oxygen delivery to body organs, poor skin health, poor performance in school, etc.

This Menstrual Coloring Book is designed to help the girl child learn the ever changing tides in her cycle with an informed mind.

***

"Wow, thank you very much. There is a Ghanaian saying; 'a man who keeps a beautiful lady for a friend is like a person who keeps a Guinea Fowl for a pet. He is likely to eat his poor pet one day," he sent her a warning wrapped in an African proverb.

"Kkkk; provided he is an excellent cook, it is fine," she replied in her usual unpredictable naughty trait.

"I am so glad I never took advantage of you. Did you know I thought of turning you into a Braii pack many times in Mpulungu? Thank you for helping me not to. You are an incredible young lady. You are funny and naughty. I will miss you daily," he thanked her for their memorable retreat to Mpulungu.

"I was vulnerable, I wanted you... but you chose not to take advantage of me. Thank you for inspiring me to see beyond the moment. You are a good man, a compassionate doctor and a gifted surgeon. I will always cherish my memories of you working late in the night on the wards and as a fish expert of Lake Tanganyika. You will always be, for me, a giant among a few good doctors," she summarized how she would remember Marx.

"These are the sweetest words I have ever heard," he expressed his sincere appreciation of her kind words.

"I am serious...," she texted him back immediately.

"If you are ever in the Tourist Capital my Lady, you remain forever my adorable Princess and I, a friend you can truly trust forever," he replied. "Happy trails to you, until we meet again. Happy trails to you, keep smiling' until then. Who cares about the clouds when we're together? Just sing a song and bring the sunny weather. Happy trails to you, 'till we meet again.

Some trails are happy ones, Others are blue. It's the way you ride the trail that counts,

Here's a happy one for you.

Happy trails to you, until we meet again.
Happy trails to you, keep smiling' until then.
Who cares about the clouds when we're together?
Just sing a song and bring the sunny weather.

Happy trails to you, 'till we meet again."

www.ingramcontent.com/pod-product-compliance
Lightning Source LLC
Chambersburg PA
CBHW070232190526
45169CB00001B/166